1992

Health Policy
and the Disadvantaged

Health Policy
and the Disadvantaged

Edited by
Lawrence D. Brown

Duke University Press
Durham and London   1991

The text of this book was originally published, in a slightly
different form and without the present index, as volume 15,
number 2 of the *Journal of Health Politics, Policy and Law*.

Library of Congress Cataloging-in-Publication Data
Health policy and the disadvantaged / edited by Lawrence D. Brown.
　　p. cm.
　Includes bibliographical references and index.
　ISBN 0-8223-1138-0 : $29.95. — ISBN 0-8223-1142-9 : $12.95
　1.Health policy—United States. 2. Handicapped—United States—
Health and hygiene. 3. Poor—United States—Health and hygiene.
I. Brown, Lawrence D. (Lawrence David), 1947–
RA395.A3H438　1991
362.1'0425—dc20　91-21831

Contents

143755

Acknowledgment

A special word of warm thanks is due to the Robert Wood Johnson Foundation for its generous support of the conference at Duke University on which this book was based. Without that support, the book could not have been published.

Health Policy
and the Disadvantaged

Introduction

Deborah A. Stone and Theodore R. Marmor

This book grows out of a conference on the disadvantaged in American health care that was sponsored by the *Journal* in the spring of 1989 and was supported by the Robert Wood Johnson Foundation and Duke University. The table of contents itself suggests a great deal about American health policymaking. The very idea of disadvantage as the focus of discussion has a 1960s ring that seems both incongruous and necessary in the 1990s. Only in America, we imagine, could—or would—a community of scholars put together a contraption such as this. By way of introduction, we want to reflect on what this social policy contraption tells us about our political souls.

The disadvantages addressed in this book are quite varied. We can play that favorite game of children's coloring books and try to group the disadvantaged by some features they share. We might see disadvantage in terms of demographic age groups—the elderly and children. We might think of it in terms of illnesses—AIDS or mental illness, or chemical dependence (to use the medical jargon for drug abuse). Or we might think of disadvantage in terms of market and governmental failure—the homeless, the hungry, and the medically uninsured all lack access to specialized markets for particular goods and services.

By whatever principle we use to classify disadvantage, we leave out some groups. Why not, as several people noted, include blacks or other ethnic groups, immigrants, the poor, the disabled, the retarded, or the chronically ill? Critics could rightly charge us with erroneous exclusion of such groups from this book, let alone from the larger policy discussion addressed. The principles, moreover, do not give us clean categories anyway. The homeless, mentally ill senior citizen and the undernourished child with AIDS both defy our attempts to locate them on our conceptual maps. These are not the exhaustive and mutually exclusive categories favored by logicians, rationalists, and mapmakers. Our purpose, however, is neither to reject nor to defend the categories. Rather, it is to show that such categorical thinking is predictably called forth by American political culture and institutions.

Unlike the health programs of Canada and much of Europe, and unlike our own public education system, American health policy has not been firmly based on universal principles. We have sequentially developed health policies designed to address the needs of groups with specific disadvantages. After World War II the progression shifted from veterans to the elderly poor (Kerr-Mills), from all the elderly (Medicare) to other groups among the poor (Medicaid), with the disabled and those with renal failure attached to Medicare in the 1970s. Such an architectural principle is guaranteed to produce growth by accretion: there will always be disadvantages, disadvantages are protean, and so there will always be new demands to incorporate new disadvantages, amoebalike. It should come as no surprise to those who spent the 1960s stretching the welfare state to meet conditions not directly confronted in the 1930s that we must now spend the 1990s making up for the omissions of the 1960s.

The structure of a society's social welfare policy is, of course, based in turn on its political ideology. By political ideology, we mean what is regarded as a legitimate sphere of action for the state and what is understood as a legitimate claim by the citizenry to mutual aid. It bears repeating that in the United States, with the exception of education, legitimacy for claims to public provision of services has never simply inhered in one's status as a member of the community. We have not developed a strong concept of what T. H. Marshall once called social citizenship rights corresponding to our rather well-developed concept of political citizenship rights.

Thus, we have had some rather strange results of political struggles over entitlements. Advocates of the poor in the 1960s and early 1970s were able to secure a legal right of otherwise eligible women to AFDC without the barrier of a one-year residency requirement. A state residency requirement, the Supreme Court held, places an undue burden on the political right of citizens to travel.[1] Advocates could not, however, persuade the Court that citizens have a right to some minimum level of subsistence.[2] To take a more current example, a federal district court in New York recently announced a right to panhandle (*New York Times* 1990). The judge saw begging as a mode of expression to be protected under the banner of freedom of speech. That we interpret begging as a voluntary act of free self-expression, rather than as an indicator of dire poverty and distress as well as a trigger to public aid, is a cruel and perverse interpretation of our political ideology. Nothing could be more emblematic of our disregard for social rights and our apotheosis of political rights than a constitutional ruling that civilized democracy requires handing out licenses to beg but not providing minimal levels of food, shelter, and medical care.

---

1. Shapiro v. Thompson, 394 U.S. 471 (1969).
2. Dandridge v. Williams, 397 U.S. 471 (1970).

For every social good except education, our social policy has rested on the distinction between attachment to and separation from the labor market. The old-age pension part of Social Security was designed to help people who did have firm attachment to the labor force to ride out their detachment once they retired. Unemployment compensation is similarly predicated on prior attachment to the work force. Even Mothers' Pensions, the precursor of AFDC, was predicated on assumptions about attachment to the labor force. In this case, though, the rationale for aid was a gendered norm that mothers should *not* enter the labor force, even if their male breadwinner had died or abandoned them.

It is quite consistent, then, that when the United States got around to establishing some kind of public guarantee of health care (through Medicare), we looked first to those who had already "earned" such a benefit by virtue of their prior participation in the work force, or in a marriage to someone in the work force. (Even though eligibility for Medicare hospital benefits turned out not to be contingent on any prior work, earnings, or contribution record, the dominant image of the elderly in the fight over Medicare was that they consisted primarily of retired workers and their spouses who had contributed FICA taxes when working. The elderly were not slouches.) Medicaid, with its grant of medical assistance on the basis of sheer poverty, was something of an unexpected anomaly. But Medicaid slid through the narrow cracks in our norms of individual self-sufficiency only by having eligibility also tied to the same family-structure criteria as AFDC or to the traditional English Poor Law categories of aged, blind, and disabled.

In a society that is deeply distrustful of public power and hesitant about redistribution, health services cannot be easily legitimized by claims about the essentialness of health, the requirement of equal treatment, or the obligations of a community to its members. We find ourselves with a plethora of categories partly because, without a dominant principle of universalism, searching out the specially needy is a mode of pressing and legitimating claims to social resources. The chapters that follow, besides providing rich descriptions of the state of health policy and politics for each of the "client" groups, illustrate the familiar mix of justifications in American politics: crisis, cost savings, and moral desert.

Virtually every one of the chapters describes a political situation in which advocates proclaim a state of crisis.[3] It is a curiosity of American political rhetoric that demonstrating or projecting a rapid rate of growth in some problem seems to command more attention than qualitative descriptions of the problem itself. Apparently, the problems are not what bother us so much as

---

3. For a striking illustration of the same tendency in public pensions, see Marmor and Mashaw (1988).

a fear that the problems are growing. The public sector, it seems, can be mobilized by threats of bigness, because we have no consensus about what constitutes badness.

The rhetoric of crisis is now very much tied to the rhetoric of cost savings. Each population of the disadvantaged is said to represent an opportunity to save money. Money spent on community-based services for the mentally ill was supposed to come from money saved on the big psychiatric institutions. Every dollar spent on prenatal care or on food aid, the advocates claimed, would reduce future medical expenses by three dollars. The bigger the crisis, the bigger the opportunity for savings. And in a world of deficits, fiscal efficiency—getting more bang for the buck—seems the one thing Americans can agree on as a worthy social goal.

Deservingness is, for Americans, the most problematic of the three classic justifications for government action in health care. There probably never was a golden age when sickness and sin were entirely different interpretations of human misfortune, and when the definition of a problem as illness carried with it an implicit judgment of innocence. But the half century between about 1920 and 1970, when the great conquest of infectious disease took place, probably came closest to such a golden era. It is no accident that the United States's belated (and limited) commitment to public health care financing was forged before the "new perspectives on health" made personal lifestyle choices a cause of disease and thus turned some sick people into sinners once again. We have only to consider AIDS to see that there is no longer a wall between sickness and sin. Because of this confusion about the moral status of the sick person, advocates for the disadvantaged are in a paradoxical position: there are political rewards for medicalizing social disadvantages (such as poverty, hunger, and addictions) and social vulnerabilities (such as old age and childhood), but there are also political dangers. Advocates have to work hard to portray their clientele either as free of any blame for their problem or as a group harmed by prior public policy and so entitled to compensatory aid.

The political logic of incremental policy expansion in health policy appears quite different in 1990 than in the spring of 1989, when the conference from which this book arises was held. Then, no one made confident predictions of the policy surprise of the 1980s—the repudiation of the so-called catastrophic addition to Medicare.

Complicated and incomplete as it was when originally enacted in 1988, the catastrophic addition to Medicare was a classic marriage of categorical thinking and interest group/government bargaining within the Washington Beltway. Never explained to the wider American public in terms they could understand and the object of shrill attack by groups that support themselves by arousing the elderly's fear of ill treatment, the catastrophic plan fell victim to one of the most extraordinary campaigns in recent American politics. Essentially, Congress became terrified that significant sectors of the elderly population would regard the redistributive financing features of the catastrophic plan as an assault on the well-being of all the elderly. And this charge stuck despite the obvious fact—obvious at least to anyone who understood what the distribution of income was like among those over 65—that only a small minority among the wealthiest of the elderly would be made financially worse off. If such confusion can dominate a relatively small sector of the health policy world, one can imagine what the fight over systematic reform of our health care arrangements would be like.

The thwarted movement towards a catastrophic addition to Medicare proceeded from the same political assumptions as do the following chapters on those who are especially disadvantaged in American medical care. Looking backward, there was the assumption that those left out—or made worse off—during the Reagan years were promising targets for moderate reforms. The Reagan fiscal revolution—combining tax cuts, military expansion, and large deficits—has driven nonincremental social policy off the agenda of American politics. As a result, all that seems possible is tinkering at the edges of current policy. On the other hand, the consequences of America's flirtation with a competitive model of health reform have left us with the worst of all possible combinations: the most expensive health care system in the world and marked dissatisfaction among patients, physicians, and payers. What is called for is serious rationalization of a system that is wrenchingly misdirected. What seems possible is a continuation of misguided incrementalism, typified in public policy discussion by talk of expanding access without changing the balance of power between providers and payers, and in corporate and health insurance circles by wishful thinking about the wonders of managed care.

America remains the most embattled site in the developed world for health policy. The chapters that follow chart the details of some of our victims, but not the shape of remedies. For that, much more than sympathy for America's unlucky will be required. And, if medical inflation continues at present rates, that pressure may be forthcoming from the board rooms of American corporations rather than from the familiar laments of American academics.

References

Marmor, T. R., and J. L. Mashaw, eds. 1988. *Social Security: Beyond the Rhetoric of Crisis*. Princeton, NJ: Princeton University Press.

New York Times. 1990. Freedom to Beg: New Law in a New Age. 30 January, p. A1.

Health Care of the Disadvantaged: The Elderly

Judith Feder

Abstract. This chapter explores threats to the maintenance and expansion of public commitment to financing health care for the elderly. Threats come from rising costs that increase financial burdens, especially on low-income elderly; efforts to contain costs that may undermine benefits; and financing initiatives that treat the elderly as the sole revenue source for addressing problems in that age group. A review of these threats provides lessons not only for sustaining and improving health care for the elderly, but also for policy toward equally or more disadvantaged groups.

Relative to other population groups considered in this volume, the elderly are decidedly advantaged. Unlike others, they are the beneficiaries of a universal, publicly financed health insurance system—Medicare—that pays their medical bills, regardless of their incomes, and assures them access to mainstream medical care. Furthermore, as a large and organized constituency that votes, the elderly are politically advantaged. That advantage is nowhere more evident than in the budget battles of the 1980s, which left Medicare and Social Security relatively unscathed while other social programs were decimated.

Political commitment to health care for the elderly does not mean the elderly are not deserving of special attention. Without government's commitment, the elderly would be sorely disadvantaged, given their considerable health care needs. And despite government's commitment, many of their needs, most especially in long-term care, go largely untouched.

However, questions about health care policy toward elderly people are somewhat different from questions asked for other disadvantaged groups. For others, the major question is whether and how to establish adequate financing for health care needs; for the elderly, the primary question is whether the current public commitment can be sustained and extended. This paper will explore that question, first by examining threats to government protection of the elderly that emerged in the 1980s, and then by considering how experience with existing programs may inhibit expansion to cover long-term care.

Despite the existence and even expansion of the Medicare program in recent years, Medicare's protection has been eroded by the continuing and growing financial burden of costs the program does not cover, by efforts to control public expenditures, and by innovations in financing—"self-financing"—that treat the elderly population as the only appropriate revenue source for solving problems in their age group.

The politics and policy associated with these developments not only have implications for Medicare's survival and improvement but also offer the following lessons, which go beyond the elderly to policy toward equally or more disadvantaged groups: (1) efforts to assure universal, non-means-tested programs should not ignore the fact that provision of adequate protection must take income into account; (2) cost containment designed to make and keep social programs affordable should be carefully designed and monitored so that preoccupation with costs does not overwhelm commitment to benefits; and (3) segmentation of the population into distinct "problem" groups should not become a segmentation of financing sources that undermines basic principles of insurance and social justice.

The financial burden of out-of-pocket expenses

Medicare was established in 1965 to assure elderly people affordable health insurance protection. Without insurance, medical costs impeded many people's access to care and constituted a sizable financial burden to those who received care. Medicare aimed to remedy these problems through a government insurance program that paid the bulk of hospital and physician bills for almost all the elderly, at rates set to reflect what hospitals cost and what physicians charged.

There is little doubt that with these policies, Medicare contributed to a marked improvement in access to care for the elderly, to the increased sophistication of that care (through support of improved technology), and (though there is more debate on this subject) to longer life expectancy for elderly people. However, Medicare never eliminated the elderly's responsibility to pay for their medical care. Beneficiaries pay a premium to finance a portion of their physician services and pay cost sharing on both physician and hospital care. As health care costs have risen (in part because of Medicare's generous policies toward provider payment), the burden of these payments has risen as well.

Increases in the burden of cost sharing under Medicare date from the beginning of the Medicare program and, for the most part, represent the unintended consequences of rising medical costs. But in the 1980s cost sharing was increased in order to reduce program costs to the federal government. The changes the Reagan administration proposed for Medicare were not the provider payment reforms that later received so much attention; rather they were proposals to shift financing from government to beneficiaries (Feder et al. 1982). Despite congressional resistance to many administration proposals, in the 1980s alone liabilities for cost sharing on services that Medicare covers more than doubled (Prospective Payment Assessment Commission 1988).

Critics of Medicare coverage have frequently observed that the elderly spend as large a share of their incomes on health care today as they did before Medicare was enacted, when spending on noncovered services as well as on cost sharing for covered services is taken into account. Those who make this observation sometimes ignore how much more (and better) health care the elderly are buying today; but they are right in emphasizing that Medicare, even supported by the welfare-based Medicaid program which pays cost sharing for the poorest elderly, has not eliminated the financial catastrophe associated with acute illness.[1]

In 1986, more than one-fifth of the elderly spent more than 15 percent of their per capita incomes out-of-pocket on medical care (not including long-term care). More than one-tenth of the elderly spent more than 20 percent of their income out-of-pocket. About half of these expenses were on services that Medicare covers. The remainder went to acute care services Medicare excludes—most notably, prescription drugs.

These out-of-pocket burdens did not go unnoticed in the 1980s. Although the early 1980s brought efforts to increase cost sharing, the late 1980s brought legislation to curtail it. In 1988, Congress passed the Medicare Catastrophic Coverage Act, touted as the largest Medicare benefit expansion since the program's enactment.

The "catastrophic" benefit initially proposed by the Reagan administration was aimed at improving Medicare coverage along the same lines as improvements in private insurance policies—that is, by setting a cap on dollars spent out-of-pocket. Congress expanded the initial administration proposal to cover a larger proportion of elderly beneficiaries and to provide coverage for prescription drugs, not previously included in Medicare, once a substantial deductible had been met. Even with the expansion, the cap can be characterized as protection against very large medical bills (roughly $2,000 in hospital and physician bills, and another $600 in prescription drug expenses).[2]

Although a minority of beneficiaries experience such large expenses (Congressional Budget Office 1988), the new benefits offer true insurance protection against the risk of very large bills that all beneficiaries face. But the catastrophic expenses described above—measured as a proportion of income—do not typically come from large medical bills. Instead they come primarily from smaller expenses by relatively low-income people. Almost all the elderly spending more than 15 percent of their income on medical bills

---

1. The following discussion draws on Feder, Moon, and Scanlon (1987).
2. The legislation had other provisions, but this discussion will focus on provisions that addressed so-called catastrophic expenditures.

had per capita incomes below $10,000. Two-thirds of them experienced "catastrophic" burdens from expenses less than $1,500 on *all* medical expenses, only some of which would even be covered under the cap. Consequently, the cap does not reduce their exposure to financial catastrophe at all (Feder, Moon, and Scanlon 1987).

This outcome reflects a continuing problem with Medicare, noted a long time ago by Davis (1975)—that is, the inequity of seemingly equal treatment in the benefit structure. While availability of Medicare to all the elderly regardless of income may constitute a political strength for the program, it may also leave the lower-income elderly inadequately protected.

The lessons from this review are twofold. First, as long as there is cost sharing, equal benefits will not provide equal protection against financial catastrophe. Income must be recognized in designing protection, as long as a program does not cover all costs. Second, a segment of the elderly population remains underinsured, despite the enactment of catastrophic protection. Protection of this population will continue to erode as health costs rise. Enhancing their protection should be kept in mind as the nation explores expansion of insurance coverage for the population under the age of 65.

The risks of cost containment

Unfortunately, the second source of erosion of Medicare benefits comes from efforts to contain cost increases that produce the growing out-of-pocket burden just described. Medicare cost-containment efforts that began in earnest in the 1980s could be applauded as a means to assure fiscal solvency for the Medicare program. Indeed, they have served in large part as a congressional alternative to administration-proposed increases in beneficiaries' financial contributions.

There is no question that rationalizing methods to pay providers is desirable, that we should move from a system in which government allows providers to determine how much they will be paid (their costs or their charges) to a system in which government makes decisions on the amount it is willing to pay. But in making that decision, government has demonstrated a willingness to assume, more than to assure, that it is setting the "right" price—that is, a price that is adequate to assure access to efficiently delivered care.

This assumption is reflected in the design of Medicare's Prospective Payment System (PPS) for hospitals.[3] PPS pays all hospitals a price per hospital case (or diagnosis) that is independent of each hospital's costs. The price is set to represent the average cost of a diagnosis across all hospitals (though distinctions are made between urban and rural hospitals and to reflect differences in geographic or other factors affecting some costs). Using the av-

---

3. The following discussion draws on Feder, Hadley, and Zuckerman (1987) and Hadley, Zuckerman, and Feder (1989).

erage means that some hospitals are paid more than costs and some are paid less. All hospitals can keep whatever profit they earn from keeping costs below the rate they are paid.

Although there is debate about the success of PPS in controlling hospital costs over time, there is little question that constraining rates and allowing profits did indeed promote a slowdown in hospital cost increases when PPS went into effect. The slowdown was particularly marked among hospitals that were paid less than their costs. Furthermore, using average costs as a payment rate created winners and losers among hospitals, thereby dividing and conquering the hospital industry as a political force and allowing Congress to constrain rate increases over time. As a result, more and more hospitals face more and more pressure to constrain their costs.

This experience is indeed a political victory for cost containment, viewed in terms of government's ability to control its spending. But from the beneficiary's perspective, the approach and experience raise some serious questions. The PPS method assumes that hospitals it "squeezes" are less efficient than the hospitals it rewards. On the surface, penalties seem to be greatest on the hospitals that are least efficient. Evidence indicates that hospitals under the greatest fiscal pressure from PPS have been hospitals with the longest lengths of stay and highest costs per case—which may be suggestive of the inefficiency PPS aims to discourage. However, it is not clear that these hospitals' higher costs are due primarily to inefficiency. PPS aims to take other costs into account by adjusting average costs for a variety of factors including local wage rates, teaching, disproportionate volume of care to the poor, and cases involving especially high costs or lengths of stay. The resulting rates are intended to represent the "fair" price for efficiently delivered care. However, adjustments are not sufficiently precise to accommodate the differences hospitals face in prices for the goods and services they must buy; nor do they even aim to adjust for other factors that can affect cost per case—specifically, differences in the severity of illness for patients with the same diagnosis and differences in the quality of care provided. Measuring these is difficult, but failure to include them in the rate calculations means that higher costs may not simply represent greater inefficiency but a difference in patients or quality of patient care.

PPS further assumes that hospitals are responding to payment constraints by increasing efficiency, rather than by reducing access or quality of care. There is some reason to question this assumption. It is not at all clear that discharging patients "sicker and quicker," as PPS encouraged, is desirable. This critique is not meant to imply that PPS is a mistake. Although it could be designed to save as much with less disruption of patterns of care,[4] its overall

---

4. See proposals for PPS reform in Feder, Hadley, and Zuckerman (1987) and Hadley, Zuckerman, and Feder (1989).

goal of limiting rate increases has merit. Rather, the goal is to highlight the risk that preoccupation with winning the battle against providers in order to control rates can override concern about the implications of expenditure control for people and care.

This tendency is not unique to PPS; it is reflected in debates about Medicare vouchers, capitated payments to so-called organized systems of care, and, most recently, methods of paying physicians. In all these areas, there is the risk that government's focus on limiting spending, rather than on achieving value for the dollar, can erode the access and quality that a public program ought to assure.

The lesson from this Medicare experience, like the lesson from cost sharing, has implications that go beyond the elderly. Efforts to promote new programs to insure the uninsured or to assist underserved groups invariably promise "innovative" financing that will keep new spending under control. This promise has become a necessary component of advocacy in an era of fiscal conservatism. But advocates must be sure that their efforts to sell fiscal responsibility will not produce mechanisms that ultimately undermine the capacity of new programs to assure access to quality care.

The limits to "self-financing"

The final source of erosion facing Medicare in the recent past relates to program financing and comes from Congress's experience with the catastrophic legislation. The financing for the new benefits in that legislation departed from traditional Medicare financing in two respects: (1) financial contributions from beneficiaries varied with their incomes, and (2) beneficiaries themselves had to bear the full costs of the benefit increase (that is, the cap).

The first change, varying costs with income, is not in itself an erosion. It may, as indicated below, represent a relatively equitable means of financing improvements in Medicare coverage. However, its introduction in conjunction with the second departure—so-called self-financing—created a political uproar that may have serious repercussions for future Medicare financing and benefit expansion.

The catastrophic benefit could have been financed with an equal premium charged to all elderly (as Secretary Bowen initially proposed). But both conservatives and liberals in Congress questioned this approach. Conservatives had come to question the desirability of Medicare's equal treatment of all beneficiaries, regardless of income and ability to pay. Relating contributions to income therefore seemed an improvement in the program. At the same time, liberals saw equal premiums as posing unequal burdens. The larger the benefit catastrophic care offered, the greater the premium would have had to be. (Estimates are that adding the full costs of the catastrophic cap would have increased the monthly Part B premium from $32 to $60 per month in 1993.)[5] For the low-income elderly, increases in the premium would have posed new and certain burdens, undermining the protection the new program was supposed to provide. Furthermore, since the higher-income elderly spend more on medical care and are more likely to reach the catastrophic cap, equal premiums would mean that revenue from the lower-income elderly would finance care to the better-off (Feder et al. 1987).

The alternative to relying on a large, equal premium was to combine a small equal premium ($4 per month in 1989) with a relatively large surcharge on income tax for the 40 percent of the elderly who pay it. The surcharge would begin at 15 percent in 1989, as some benefits were introduced, and rise to 28 percent by 1993, when all benefits were in place. There would also be a cap on payments, set at $800 in 1989 ($1,050 in 1993), for individuals whose gross incomes exceeded $42,000, a level of payment that would be reached by approximately 10 percent of the elderly. The maximum was estimated to equal about six times the value of the fully implemented benefit (Congressional Budget Office 1988)—a benefit that many of the better-off elderly already had through private insurance at much lower (or, if their previous employer paid it, even zero) cost.

However, the premise on which Congress enacted the legislation—that the benefits were sufficiently attractive to the elderly to support the change in financing—was unfounded. Organizations of the elderly and legislators who listened to them misread their constituency. Reading it accurately, however, is not a simple proposition. Some interpret the reaction of the elderly community as a desire to have someone else pay for the benefits they receive. If that is correct, this attitude poses a major threat to financing future Medicare benefits, most especially for long-term care, where contributions from the elderly are likely to be fiscally as well as politically essential.

An alternative point of view is that it is not the contribution, or even the income-related nature of the contribution, that is causing so much trouble. Rather, it is the introduction of income-related financing in the context of "self-financing" (and on a benefit perceived as having relatively little value, especially to those who pay the most) that has caused the elderly to rebel. Having the elderly with higher incomes contribute more to financing is not the same as saying the elderly are fully responsible for financing care to their own age group and that all resources and redistribution associated with the new benefits must come from within that age group.

The latter premise, on which the catastrophic legislation rested, would not only make it impossible to expand Medicare benefits to long-term care (there

---

5. Letter from Dan Rostenkowski, chairman, Committee on Ways and Means, U.S. House of Representatives, 6 December 1988.

just isn't enough money there); it also undermines basic concepts of social justice. Redistributing income to assist those who cannot afford to assist themselves is a societal responsibility. If it is segmented by age group, it threatens our capacity to pool the nation's resources to deal with a myriad of social problems—including, but by no means limited to, long-term care.

Expanding Medicare's protection: Long-term care

Although the elderly may be somewhat advantaged when it comes to insurance for health care, they are decidedly disadvantaged when it comes to their need for long-term care.[6] Long-term care is a financial as well as an emotional catastrophe. But we do not treat it as we do other financial disasters. Private insurance has been virtually nonexistent for long-term care (though, as described below, it is now beginning to emerge); and government finances long-term care (through the welfare-based Medicaid program) only after people have exhausted their resources (or if they had none to begin with). Although this mechanism of government support is important in assuring access to needed care, it does not protect against financial catastrophe; it protects only after catastrophe has occurred.

There is growing consensus that victim-based financing for long-term care ought to be replaced with financing that spreads the risk beyond victims—in other words, with insurance. However, there is considerable debate about whether the primary provider of insurance should be the public or the private sector. Advocates of private insurance argue that despite the lack of private long-term care insurance in the past, private insurance can develop and can offer a substantial population the protection they need. However, a strong case can be made that the factors that have inhibited insurers in the past will limit the value or scope of private insurance in the future; and that, consequently, social insurance is the most appropriate approach to long-term care financing.

Private insurers' reluctance to enter the long-term care market reflects the financial risk that claims costs will exceed premium revenues. The risks are that only persons likely to use services will buy insurance (adverse selection); that once insured, people will overstate their disability and use more services than they would have without insurance (moral hazard); and that increases in service prices between the time insurance is purchased and the time it is used (which could easily exceed ten years in long-term care) will produce costs greater than anticipated.

Although long-term care policies have grown dramatically in recent years (from almost zero five years ago to about a million today), insurance products now in effect are designed to protect insurers against these risks, thereby re-

---

6. The following discussion draws on Feder and Scanlon 1988, 1989.

ducing protection offered to consumers. Initial policies (which constitute the bulk of the million policies now in force) protected insurers by excluding coverage for certain conditions (like Alzheimer's disease), emphasizing institutional rather than in-home services, requiring prior receipt of skilled (e.g., nursing) care rather than personal care. Newer policies have eliminated many of these restrictions. However, their premiums are higher, reducing the number of elderly who can afford them.

Furthermore, they share with earlier policies three critical limitations. First, and not surprising, policies are not sold to persons who are already impaired or are very old. Second, benefits are for the most part specified in fixed-dollar terms. A person aged 65 could buy a policy that pays $50 per day, almost the full cost of a nursing home today. But that person may not need nursing home care for twenty years, by which time $50 would cover only a small portion of nursing home costs. Although additional inflation protection can be purchased, it substantially increases the annual premium (by about 25 percent). Third, although many states prohibit insurers from raising insurance premiums for specific individuals, insurers are allowed to raise premiums (or cancel policies) for whole groups of insured, if financial experience warrants. The result could be that people who have paid premiums for years could be unable to afford to continue payments. Not only would they be without protection; their payments would be forgone.

Insurers are well aware of the limitations in marketing long-term care insurance to the over-65 population. Although they have by no means abandoned that market, many companies have turned their attention to an alternative marketing strategy—selling long-term care insurance through employment, rather than to individuals. Selling this way could reduce the risks of adverse selection and would allow individuals, by buying at younger ages, to contribute smaller amounts over time to cover the high costs of future benefits.

Although some believe the employer-based market can grow substantially, particularly if afforded the favorable tax treatment health care benefits now receive, employers' growing dissatisfaction with the costs of existing health care benefits, especially for retirees, raises questions about their likely interest in moving into long-term care. Some companies have been willing to offer long-term care insurance to their employees, but almost none have been willing to contribute toward their employees' premiums.

Alongside enthusiasm for the growth of private long-term care insurance, then, there is growing recognition that substantial numbers of elderly, now and in the future, are unlikely to receive adequate protection from that source. Even if private long-term care insurance grows, a substantial minority of the elderly will be unable to afford it, and even those covered by policies may remain subject to considerable financial risk.

In these circumstances a strong argument can be made for social insurance as the appropriate mechanism for financing long-term care. Social insurance spreads the risk over the largest population and over time, insures the already impaired as well as the healthy, and allows for an equitable distribution of burdens and costs across income groups. And, recent Medicare experience notwithstanding, government is likely to find it more difficult than a private business would to walk away from even an expensive commitment to provide benefits.

However, Medicare experience and fiscal concerns place a significant barrier to making that commitment in the first place. Furthermore, experience with the catastrophic legislation has given Congress some pause about adding new benefits for the elderly. Given the high costs of a long-term care program (in the neighborhood of $60 billion per year for comprehensive benefits), as well as the high costs of existing benefits, the elderly would indeed be expected to contribute to long-term care financing. If, as some congressmen believe, the backlash against the catastrophic legislation indicates an unwillingness to make that contribution, expanded government support of long-term care becomes highly unlikely.

The primary caregivers of the impaired elderly are, after all, their children, who would share their concern about the costs of long-term care. Polls indicate that people of all ages and all income groups are far more supportive of government intervention in long-term care—where even the better-off lack protection—than they are for expanding health insurance protection to the currently uninsured.[7]

As elsewhere, it is difficult to predict how the politics of long-term care issues will play out. However, should we move in the direction of social insurance, or even expanded public financing that falls somewhat short of that concept, the lessons from the Medicare experience, outlined above, are clearly relevant. If we pursue universal insurance protection, we must be mindful that concern with equal protection regardless of income does not obscure the special problems of the poor and better-off; that concern with containing costs does not lead us to underfund benefits; and that concern with fiscal fairness across population groups and generations does not undermine our commitment to pool the nation's resources to help those who are unable to help themselves.

References

Congressional Budget Office. 1988. The Medicare Catastrophic Coverage Act of 1988. Staff working paper.

Davis, Karen. 1975. Equal Treatment and Unequal Benefits: The Medicare Program. *Milbank Memorial Fund Quarterly* 53 (4): 449–88.

---

7. "The American Public Views Long-Term Care," a survey of 1,000 registered voters conducted in July 1987 by RL Associates, Princeton, NJ.

Feder, Judith, Jack Hadley, and Stephen Zuckerman. 1987. How Did Medicare's Prospective Payment System Affect Hospitals? *New England Journal of Medicine* 317: 867–73.

Feder, Judith, John Holahan, Randall Bovbjerg, and Jack Hadley. 1982. Health. In *The Reagan Experiment*, ed. John Palmer and Isabel Sawhill. Washington, DC: The Urban Institute Press.

Feder, Judith, Marilyn Moon, and William Scanlon. 1987. Medicare Reform: Nibbling at Catastrophic Costs. *Health Affairs* 6 (4): 5–19.

Feder, Judith, and William Scanlon. 1988. Synthesis of Reports on Reforms in Long-Term Care Financing. Washington, DC: Georgetown University Center for Health Policy Studies (working paper no. 850-1).

———. 1989. Problems and Prospects in Financing Long-Term Care. In *Care and Cost: Current Issues in Health Policy*, ed. Kenneth McLennan and Jack Meyer. Boulder, CO: Westview Press.

Hadley, Jack, Stephen Zuckerman, and Judith Feder. 1989. Profits and Fiscal Pressure in the Prospective Payment System: Their Impacts on Hospitals. *Inquiry* 26 (Fall).

Prospective Payment Assessment Commission. 1988. *Medicare Prospective Payment and the American Health Care System: Report to the Congress*. Washington, DC: ProPAC.

Rich, Spencer. 1989. Medicare Coalition Shaken by Its Own Handiwork. *Washington Post*, 27 July, pp. A1, A17 (estimates of the Joint Committee on Taxation, U.S. House of Representatives).

Child Health Policy in the U.S.: The Paradox of Consensus

Alice Sardell

Abstract. This examination of child health policy begins by reviewing the politics of maternal and child health services from the early twentieth century to the Reagan administration, including the role of feminist movements, the development of pediatrics, and the expansion of federal involvement during the 1960s. Next, the politics of Medicaid expansion as a strategy for addressing child health issues are discussed and current critiques of child health services in the U.S. examined, along with proposals to restructure health care financing and delivery. Central to the politics of child health policy during the 1980s and into the 1990s is the way in which child health has been defined. Infant mortality and childhood illness are presented as preventable problems. Investment in young children is discussed as a prudent as well as a compassionate policy, one which will reduce future health care costs and enhance our position in the international economy. Unlike other "disadvantaged groups," children are universally viewed as innocent and deserving of societal support. Framing child health issues in these terms helped to produce consensus on the expansion of Medicaid eligibility. Other issues involve the restructuring of health care financing and delivery, however, and on these issues conflict is far more likely than consensus.

Introduction

Child health is an area in which the paradoxes of American health policy are very clear. We provide excellent, high-technology, specialized services to those with acute conditions while we neglect primary care and the social factors that increase medical risk. The U.S. ranks first in the world in its ability

The author wishes to thank Sara Rosenbaum for generously sharing her manuscript on child health policy and for her helpful comments on this article. Elizabeth Fogarty of the National Commission to Prevent Infant Mortality and Katherine Kiedrowski of the National Association of Community Health Centers were also very generous in sharing their knowledge of the intricacies of legislation related to maternal and child health services. James Morone's comments on this paper in its conference form were very useful. The author would also like to acknowledge Miriam Pope's contribution to this article.

to save the lives of premature and very small infants, yet ranks fifteenth in the proportion of babies born at low birthweight (Schorr 1988: 66). (Low birthweight is defined as 2,500 grams or less and is an important risk factor for neonatal and postneonatal[1] infant mortality, for morbidity during the first year of life, and for mental and physical disability later in life [Starfield 1985: 525].)

In terms of infant mortality (death between birth and age 1), the U.S. rate was the highest of 21 industrial nations in 1986, at 10.4 per 1,000 births. The black rate was twice that of the white rate (House Select Committee 1988: 38). As stated in shocking terms by the National Commission to Prevent Infant Mortality, unless the present infant mortality rate is reduced, we will lose more infants between 1988 and 2000 than the total number of battlefield deaths of Americans in World War I, World War II, Korea, and Vietnam combined (National Commission 1988: 8).

Our infant mortality rate has become worse during the twentieth century in comparison to the rates of other countries. In 1918, the U.S. Children's Bureau found that the U.S. infant mortality rate was sixth among 20 countries; in 1986 it was thirteenth among these same 20 nations and eighteenth world-wide. It is not just among the black population that our infant mortality rate compares negatively with other nations. The white infant mortality rate in the U.S. is the same as the overall rate of Spain and Singapore. Our white infant mortality rate considered alone would rank the U.S. tenth worldwide. Our black infant mortality rate considered alone makes us twenty-eighth in the world—the same ranking as Costa Rica, Portugal, and Poland, and lower than Greece, Cuba, Czechoslovakia, and Bulgaria (CDF 1989: 12).

U.S. vaccination rates for young children have declined since 1980, while the incidence of major childhood illness has increased. More than one-fifth of all two-year-olds were not fully immunized against polio, rubella, mumps, or measles in 1985. Our immunization rates for DPT (diphtheria, pertussis, tetanus) among children under age 1 are half that of Western Europe, including Spain and Italy, and Canada and Israel (OTA 1988: 142–43).

What is so ironic, of course, is that we spend a larger proportion of our national GNP on health care than does any other country in the world—11.1 percent in 1987.

The effective communication of this kind of data, along with the argument that the rate of infant mortality and childhood illness and disability could be reduced, produced a consensus among policymakers in the mid-1980s that action had to be taken to improve the health of American children. One consequence of that consensus was a series of legislative provisions which have

---

1. Neonatal infant mortality is death up to 27 days; postneonatal infant mortality includes deaths from 28 days to one year.

expanded eligibility for Medicaid and separated it from eligibility for Aid to Families with Dependent Children (AFDC), to which it had been linked since Medicaid's inception.

We are now in a new phase of agenda building/policy formulation in which the central question is, What should be done about child health beyond making more people eligible for Medicaid? One set of proposals is to increase employer and/or government financing of maternal and child health services. Another aspect of the policy discussion is the importance of lifestyle issues and the physical and social environment in the birth and growth of healthy children. Yet, unlike those who argued in the 1970s that the "limits of medicine" implied that there should be less health care (Knowles 1977), those concerned with child health today would argue for more health services, but would define health care more broadly. The National Institute of Medicine and the National Commission to Prevent Infant Mortality both recommend the provision of services that address social factors that impact on health status—nutrition counseling, substance abuse treatment, parenting education, etc. This is a model of health services in which medical care is tightly integrated with educational and social service.

This model for improving the health of mothers and children is not new— it goes back to the child welfare movement of the Progressive era. It is a model to which some of the health policy community returned in the mid-1960s when federal community and migrant health centers were initially funded, and is again being discussed at the end of the 1980s by those concerned with child health issues.

Policy formulation will now, however, be more complicated and problematic than it was when Medicaid expansion was the issue in the mid-1980s. Some of the current proposals involve major changes in the financing and structure of the health system. Their implementation would force policymakers to confront the broader issue of the extent to which the nation will invest in "human capital" when there is great concern about trade and budget deficits. As these issues emerge, the "consensus" about child health may begin to unravel. There are indications that this process may have already begun.

In the first section of this chapter I review government activity related to maternal and child health services during the twentieth century, focusing on themes relevant to child health policy today. Next, I describe the politics of the expansion of Medicaid eligibility at the federal level, and briefly discuss the limits of Medicaid expansion as a policy for increasing access to health services. I then analyze the way that child health issues have been framed during the 1980s. Such an analysis can help to explain why prenatal care and child health services have drawn so much attention lately, and paradoxically, why the way in which the issues have been defined may be problematic for future policymaking. Next, I summarize the current critiques of U.S. maternal and child health services and the proposals that have been made to change them, including legislative action on such proposals during the 101st Congress. Finally, I speculate on the future of child health policy in the U.S. by analyzing the constituencies that could be mobilized to support broad change and the structural and political constraints that could impede such change.

Limits of time and space preclude my dealing with crucial policy issues relating to the care and treatment of chronically or severely ill or disabled children, such as the financing of the catastrophic costs of children's illness. The focus here will be on the prenatal, preventive, and primary care services which, according to the community of child health experts, can reduce our high infant mortality rate and prevent much childhood illness and lifelong disability.

Child health policy at the federal level: From the Progressive era to the Reagan "revolution"

Child health advocacy in the Progressive era.   One of the issues addressed by the social reformers of the Progressive period was the welfare of children, particularly poor children. Industrialization and large-scale immigration to the U.S. produced high rates of infectious disease and death in infants and young children. Children worked in factories, lived in inadequate housing, and suffered from malnutrition (Black 1988: 213; Wilson 1989: 28–29).

Diarrhea was a major cause of infant death, and one of the first efforts made to reduce infant mortality was the establishment of infant milk stations to provide inexpensive sterilized milk in urban working-class areas. In 1908 the New York City Bureau of Child Hygiene was established, the first in the nation. The bureau sent nurses to visit new babies and to teach their mothers how to care for them. It also provided health exams to children in the public schools (Halpern 1988: 84; Wilson 1989: 30). At the national level, activities that focused on child welfare included the first White House conference on children in 1908, the birth of the American Association for the Prevention of Infant Mortality in 1910, and the establishment of the U.S. Children's Bureau in 1912 (Halpern 1988: 74).

Most of the child health activists in private welfare organizations and in government agencies were women. Women's groups, such as the League of Women Voters and the Women's Joint Congressional Committee, worked with health activists for the passage of the Maternity and Infancy (Shepphard-Towner) Act of 1921, legislation which provided federal matching funds to states to establish prenatal and child health services (Black 1988: 217; Wilson 1989: 40). Opponents of the legislation included the American Medical Association (AMA), chiropractors, and those opposed to women's suffrage. During the debate, members of Congress made antifeminist remarks and the AMA labeled the act as "socialistic." Women's magazines were very supportive of the legislation, and the potential votes of newly enfranchised women were a major factor in its passage (Black 1988: 217–24; Wilson 1989: 38–42).

The Shepphard-Towner Act was the first grant-in-aid program in health. Shepphard-Towner funds were used to establish 3,000 clinics where women physicians and public health nurses examined children and taught their mothers and older sisters (in "little mothers" classes) about infant care, nutrition, and childhood illness (Black 1988: 217–18). The renewal of the Shepphard-Towner legislation after five years was actively opposed by the AMA and the Catholic church. Congress voted in 1927 to extend the legislation for two years and then to repeal it (Wilson 1989: 46–47).

Three aspects of child health advocacy in the first part of the twentieth century are noteworthy. First, women physicians who established maternal and child health programs incorporated the values of the female-dominated popular health movement of the nineteenth century by emphasizing the education of mothers, preventive services such as immunization and nutrition counseling, and work in the community (such as "family visitors") as well as the clinic. Second, these health activists avoided direct competition with general practitioners by not providing treatment for illness (Black 1988: 214–16, 219). Third, pediatricians had a special relationship to the child health movement, which was quite different from that of most general practitioners and the AMA.

Pediatrics and the child welfare movement. Pediatrics began to develop as a specialty during the second half of the nineteenth century, primarily as a separate academic area. A section on diseases of children was created by the AMA in 1879, and the American Pediatric Society was founded in 1888 (Wilson 1989: 28). Pediatricians worked in the child welfare movement, providing it with greater legitimacy and using it to support their own demands for the recognition of pediatrics as a unique medical specialty (see Halpern 1988: 74–75). Pediatrics, unlike most medical specialties, defined itself as providing preventive and primary care, focusing on issues of normal development rather than pathology. This is uncommon within American medicine. Yet by the 1930s, the majority of pediatricians, like other American physicians, were private practitioners and provided such primary care services mainly to the middle class.

The child health clinics established in the 1920s offered "well-baby conferences," in which health professionals evaluated children's growth and development and advised mothers on many aspects of child rearing. Such services were promoted by the Children's Bureau and national child health organizations, and a demand for them was generated among middle-class as well as working-class mothers. At the same time, one group of pediatricians campaigned to restrict the use of clinics to families unable to pay for private pediatric care (Halpern 1988: 85–87, 91, 93, 99–100). A specialty which was nurtured by a social movement to improve the health of poor mothers and children had become privatized.

Pediatricians, however, continued to be active on social policy issues. During the 1930s (male) pediatricians replaced feminist activists in policy positions in government and private sector organizations concerned with children's health (Black 1988: 225).

The Depression and World War II.   The Shepphard-Towner Act expired just as the Depression began, and states were unable to provide maternal and child health care (Wilson 1989: 49). While proposals for comprehensive health insurance were excluded from the Roosevelt administration's draft of the Social Security bill because of the opposition of the AMA (Stevens 1971: 188, 190), Shepphard-Towner was reborn as Title V of the Social Security Act of 1935. Title V was to be administered by the Children's Bureau and included funds for maternal and child health services and for identifying and treating conditions that could result in crippling (Wilson 1989: 52).

Until the beginning of World War II, Title V primarily funded programs for planning, training, and preventive health projects. Little direct medical care was provided. However, during World War II, the Children's Bureau administered a separate program of prenatal and obstetrical care for the wives of servicemen, the Emergency Maternity and Infant Care Program. This was the largest tax-supported medical care program ever funded solely by the federal government (ibid.: 53–54). Opposition to the expansion of publicly funded medical care was deflected by labeling it as an emergency program and by limiting it to the wives of servicemen in the lowest pay grades. One and a half million women received care under the Emergency Maternity and Infant Care Program, and although maternal and child health programs were again limited to preventive health services after 1949, a precedent had been established for providing federally funded prenatal, obstetrical, and postpartum care (Davis and Schoen 1978: 123–24; Marieskind 1980: 93–94).

The expansion of child health services during the 1960s.   During the 1960s, when the role of the federal government in social policy was broadened, low-income women and children became the beneficiaries of more extensive health financing and health services programs. Medicare was passed in 1965 after a fourteen-year effort, and with it, Medicaid (Title XIX of the Social Security Act). Medicaid provided federal funds to the states on a cost-sharing basis to pay for medical services for the poor. Both Medicare and Medicaid were financing programs which were to pay for health services delivered primarily by the private sector. Medicaid became the major source of public funding for children's health services.

As early as 1966, the Department of Health, Education and Welfare (DHEW) proposed that state Medicaid agencies take direct responsibility for providing preventive health services to children of low-income families, a responsibility not being fulfilled by private practitioners. This proposal became the Early Periodic Screening Diagnosis and Treatment Program (EPSDT), enacted by Congress as part of the Social Security Amendments of 1967. States were required to screen all Medicaid-eligible children for potentially handicapping conditions and then to arrange treatment for conditions which were found (Goggin 1987: 52–55). Advocates for the EPSDT program hoped that the program would be structured to bring together all children's health services (ibid.: 54), but this was not done. Children's health services continued to be provided by several different federal programs which were not coordinated with related social service programs for children. The Children's Bureau lost most of its programs to other bureaus within DHEW in 1967.[2] Title V programs came under the jurisdiction of the Public Health Service (Wilson 1989: 54–55).

In 1965, as part of the War on Poverty, the federal government funded a small demonstration project with the goal of increasing access of the poor to health care and providing a model of comprehensive, community-based care. The first group of "neighborhood health centers" were to provide health services to the population of a specific geographical area and to serve as a center for community organization and economic development. The health care provided was not to be limited to clinical medicine but was to involve concepts of social medicine, including intervention in the physical and social environment (nutrition and food supply, housing, sewerage, etc.) of the population being served. In addition, community residents were to be trained and employed at the center and were to participate in its governance. By 1971, 150 centers had been funded. In 1975, these programs received their own separate legislative authority and were renamed "community health centers." The 1975 legislation limited the extent to which nontraditional community health services could be provided, and in the same year, DHEW initiated a policy shift from the funding of a small number of comprehensive health centers based on the original social medicine model to the funding of a larger number of small projects providing basic medical services.

During the Carter administration funding for this program was increased so that by 1981 there were more than 800 community health centers. However, four-fifths of them were small rural and urban health projects. The expansion of this program, and that of the National Health Service Corps, which had been established in 1970 to provide doctors and other health professionals to medically underserved areas, was part of an effort by the Public Health Service

---

2. The Children's Bureau, which had originally been located in the Department of Labor, was transferred to the Federal Security Agency in 1946. That agency became the Department of Health, Education and Welfare in 1953 (Wilson 1989: 54).

during the Carter years to "fill in the gaps" in the health service delivery structure. Most of the population served by community health centers are women and children (Sardell 1988).

Also during the Democratic administrations of the 1960s, federally funded maternal and child health and family planning programs were expanded. Amendments to Title V of the Social Security Act authorized funding for comprehensive health care projects in low-income areas which would provide prenatal and postpartum care to women and dental and medical services to children. In 1967, Congress specified that family planning services for low-income women be provided under Title V and three years later passed the Family Planning Services and Population Research Act, which authorized additional funds to provide family planning services. Several nutrition programs for children were enacted during the 1960s as well, including the Women, Infants, and Children (WIC) Program, which provides nutrition counseling and nutritious food to pregnant and lactating women and to children up to age 5.

The impact of federal programs.   The health financing and health care delivery programs initiated by the federal government in the 1960s clearly increased access to care for low-income pregnant women and children. The proportion of women seeking care in their first trimester of pregnancy increased during the period 1969–1980. This was especially true for black women. In 1969, 43 percent of black women initiated care in the first trimester of their pregnancy; in 1980, 63 percent of black women did so (Institute of Medicine 1988: 49). Children with Medicaid use more medical care than children from low-income families without public health insurance (OTA 1988: 55–56).

There is also evidence that publicly funded reproductive, maternal, and child health services have helped to reduce mortality and morbidity among children. Multivariate regression analysis of the relationship between health care resources and neonatal mortality (up to four weeks of life) done at the county level found that reductions in neonatal mortality in the 1960s and 1970s were related to the introduction of neonatal intensive care services, the legalization of abortion, the availability of family planning services, and, especially for blacks, Medicaid coverage of prenatal care. Reductions in postneonatal mortality (deaths from one month to one year), which are usually the result of accidents or infectious disease rather than birth defects, were found at the county level to be related to higher levels of medical expenditures, higher pediatrician-to-population ratios, and the presence of a community health center. Historically, postneonatal mortality has declined in periods when access to health services has increased. Postneonatal mortality rates declined in the 1930s and 1940s, but the rate of decline slowed in the 1950s with the end of the federal Emergency Maternity and Infant Care Program. A large decline occurred in the late 1960s, when more public funding was provided for reproductive, maternal, and child health programs. Since 1970 the rate of decline has again slowed, and in some time periods in the 1970s and 1980s there was no reduction in postneonatal mortality at all (Starfield 1985: 530–32).

A variety of studies in the U.S. also indicate that access to health services reduces the severity of illness in children with bacterial meningitis, asthma, and diabetes (ibid.: 534–39). The rates of rheumatic fever, an illness which can be prevented by treating strep infections, declined by 60 percent in areas of Baltimore with a community health center but did not decline in similar areas of the same city that did not have a health center (Geiger 1984: 29).

Retrenchment in federal spending for maternal and child health services.
While the first ten years of the Medicaid program was a period of expansion in eligibility and benefits, the second decade was, particularly for children's health services, a period of retrenchment. During the latter part of the 1970s, inflation rates were almost as high as increases in program expenditures, so that the actual availability of services increased very little. Beginning in 1972, there was a shift within Medicaid away from spending on health services for nondisabled children as a higher proportion of Medicaid funds went to pay for services for aged, blind, and disabled Supplemental Security Income recipients. In 1972, 18 percent of all Medicaid expenditures paid for services for nondisabled children under age 21; in 1987 the proportion was 13 percent. Although Medicaid is the major source of funding for children's health services, almost three-quarters of all Medicaid expenditures are spent on services for the aged, blind, and disabled. While nondisabled children and their parents constituted 66 percent of all Medicaid recipients in 1987, their health services accounted for only 25 percent of Medicaid expenditures in that year (Oberg and Polich 1988: 85–88).

In the early part of the 1980s, Medicaid funding and funding for federal grant programs in health were cut as part of the Reagan administration's efforts to reduce spending for social programs and to return fiscal and administrative responsibility for welfare and health policy to the states. The Omnibus Budget Reconciliation Act of 1981 reduced the federal government's share of Medicaid for three years and changed the eligibility rules for the program so that 440,000 poor working families lost their Medicaid coverage (ibid.: 87). It also repealed penalties for states not complying with the requirements of the EPSDT program (Rosenbaum 1988a: 21).

These reductions in federal spending for Medicaid were accompanied by the creation of block grants to the states to replace categorical health services programs. Seven categorical grant programs for children's health services became part of the Maternal and Child Health Block Grant. Block grants were funded at lower levels than the previous total funding for the separate categorical grants (Kimmich 1985: 21). Funding for maternal and child health programs was reduced by 18 percent and the Community Health Center Program, which became the Primary Care Block Grant, had its funds cut 24 percent from the fiscal year 1981 level. In addition, the Omnibus Budget Reconciliation Act of 1981 eliminated the mandated Title V comprehensive maternity and infant care programs, children and youth projects, and family planning and dental services programs initiated in the 1960s (Rosenbaum 1988a: 21–22).

When inflation is considered, federal funding for maternal and child health programs, community health centers, and migrant health centers decreased by 32 percent between 1978 and 1984, and Medicaid spending per child declined by 13 percent. During this same time period the proportion of babies born to families with incomes below the poverty level increased from 18 to 24 percent (OTA 1988: 7). In response to these federal cuts, most states reduced maternal and child health services (Rosenbaum et al. 1988: 318).

These reversals in the growth of spending for reproductive, maternal, and child health services and subsequent evidence of the unmet need for these services was a stimulus for new policy initiatives in the area of child health in the mid-1980s. It is to the politics of these initiatives that I now turn.

Child health on the policy agenda in the 1980s: The expansion of Medicaid eligibility

Child health was again on the policy agenda in the late 1970s and throughout the 1980s as part of a more general focus on "children's issues" (*National Journal* 1988: 2934–39). In 1979, the U.S. Surgeon General's report had called the reduction of infant mortality a "fundamental national goal" (OTA 1988: 5), but in the early 1980s it became clear that the nation was moving away from realizing that goal. Beginning in 1984, Congress enacted a series of reforms that increased the number of pregnant women and children eligible for the Medicaid program and separated Medicaid from the AFDC program to which it had long been linked. These changes made Medicaid a separate "public health program with its own financial eligibility standards and entry points" (Rosenbaum 1988a: 37).

Sara Rosenbaum, who was from 1983 to 1988 the health policy director of the Children's Defense Fund (CDF), has written a book on child health policy in which she chronicles the politics of the Medicaid expansions of the 1980s. Rosenbaum contrasts the unsuccessful attempt to expand eligibility and services under the EPSDT program for children in the late 1970s with the Medicaid expansions in the mid-1980s. The Carter administration's Child Health Assessment Program (CHAP) failed to be enacted by Congress between 1977 and 1980 because of state opposition to federal sanctions in the legislation, the failure of child advocacy groups to use the media to arouse the public on children's health issues, antiabortion amendments added to the CHAP bills, opposition by conservative members of Congress (Rosenbaum 1988a: 12–16), and the "lack of a perceived crisis" (ibid.: 16). In the mid-1980s, child advocacy groups and congressional committees reached the press and the public with information about a crisis in child health and worked with a broad coalition of state officials, interest groups, and members of Congress to expand eligibility for the Medicaid program (ibid.: 25–36).

The years in which funding was decreased for Medicaid and maternal and child health and nutrition programs were years of economic recession and increased unemployment. Stories about increases in the numbers of poor pregnant women and malnourished and sick children were reported in the media. In 1983, House and Senate Democrats began to work on expanding eligibility for Medicaid. At the same time officials in southern states, where infant mortality was the highest, became interested in new initiatives in maternal and child health. This interest was stimulated in part by the work of CDF and other child advocacy groups at the state level (ibid.: 23).

The February 1983 vote to establish the Select Committee on Children, Youth and Families in the House of Representatives was a significant step in focusing public attention and congressional action on children's issues. The large affirmative vote, coming after years of effort by Congressman George Miller of California, reflected the forces that would put children's issues on the governmental agenda. Congress was responding to reports about the impact of cuts in social programs on families, the existence of women as a voting block concerned about these issues (the votes of newly enfranchised women had been the catalyst for enactment of the Shepphard-Towner Act in 1921), and the mobilization of a policy community of interest groups and liberal members of Congress focused on children and families (*New York Times* 1983: A18). The select committee held a series of hearings in various parts of the country on the relationship between low birthweight and access to prenatal care (*National Journal* 1986a: 2257).

During 1984, the CDF and the Food Research and Action Center issued studies on the state of child health in the U.S. which received wide publicity and congressional attention. The CDF documented a large increase in poor children as well as a decrease in the proportion of women receiving late or no prenatal care. At the same time, the Southern Governors Association appointed a Task Force on Infant Mortality, which in 1985 recommended that states have the option to provide Medicaid to pregnant women and children with family incomes below the federal poverty level (Rosenbaum 1988a: 26–27, 30–31, 36).

Provisions included in the Deficit Reduction Act of 1984 mandated that states provide Medicaid for all pregnant women and children under age 5 with family incomes meeting the eligibility criteria for AFDC, even if they were in families which did not meet other AFDC criteria, in having, for example, two parents present (*Congressional Quarterly* 1989d: 965). This was a "decoupling" of Medicaid from AFDC, making the 1965 Ribicoff amendment, which had been optional for the states, mandatory.

A broad coalition of groups worked to enact this legislation, including the Children's Defense Fund, the American Academy of Pediatrics, the March of Dimes, the National Association of Community Health Centers, the Association of Maternal and Child Health Programs, the Catholic Conference, and the National Governors Association. Conservative, right-to-life members of Congress and some corporate business leaders also were supportive (Rosenbaum 1988a: 32–33). The CDF and the Catholic Conference, along with key congressional staff, had previously negotiated a separation of child health issues from the abortion issue (ibid.: 28).

Subsequent expansions of Medicaid eligibility were enacted as part of the budget reconciliation process. New provisions would initially be state options and in later legislation were federally mandated. In some ways, the budget reconciliation process has been helpful to child health advocates. Reconciliation rules limit the number of amendments that can be offered on a budget bill, and in a very large piece of legislation, such as the budget bills, controversial provisions have less time to be considered (*National Journal* 1989: 580).

The next set of Medicaid reforms were provisions of the 1986 and 1987 Omnibus Budget Reconciliation Acts. The Omnibus Budget Reconciliation Act of 1986 allowed states to disregard assets in determining Medicaid eligibility for pregnant women and for children under age 5, and to grant automatic eligibility to pregnant women while their applications were being processed and for 60 days after they gave birth. It also allowed states to provide Medicaid coverage to pregnant women and to infants and to phase in Medicaid coverage for children up to age 8 in families with incomes between the AFDC eligibility level and the federal poverty level. The Omnibus Budget Reconciliation Act of 1987 allowed states to cover all pregnant women and infants with family incomes up to 185 percent of the poverty level. In 1988, as part of the Medicare Catastrophic Coverage Act, Congress mandated that by 1990 state Medicaid programs cover all pregnant women and infants who have family incomes which do not exceed 100 percent of the federal poverty level. This legislation did not have a great impact because 30 states have already expanded eligibility to cover pregnant women and infants with family incomes up to 100 percent of the poverty level, and 10 other states cover pregnant women and children whose family incomes are above the federal poverty level (Rosenbaum memo 1988b: III 17–28).

The impetus for these Medicaid expansions came from a series of 1985 studies by congressional committees, the Children's Defense Fund, and the Institute of Medicine, which got wide media coverage. These expansions in eligibility were again supported by a broad coalition of state officials, child advocacy and women's groups, and members of Congress (Rosenbaum 1988a: 34–39).

The limitations of the Medicaid expansions

While the Medicaid reforms of the 1980s have reduced the financial barriers to health care for numbers of poor pregnant women and infants, there are still major obstacles to access for these populations and for other poor children.

In terms of Medicaid itself, the 1988 mandate that all pregnant women with incomes below the federal poverty level be eligible for Medicaid by 1990 still leaves large numbers of women uninsured for prenatal care. These are most likely to be young, black, or Hispanic women and women working in the service or retail sectors of the economy. In 1987, more than a quarter (26 percent) of all women of childbearing age had no insurance for prenatal care (IOM 1988: 62). One-third of all U.S. births are to women with incomes less than 150 percent of the poverty level (ibid.: 66).

The expansion of Medicaid eligibility to children up to age 8 in families with incomes below the poverty level is not mandatory for the states, and some states will not opt to expand coverage. While children in families with incomes up to 200 percent of the poverty level are unlikely to be covered by private health insurance, many states provide Medicaid to older children only if their family incomes are well below the poverty level. The reforms in the enrollment process made for pregnant women and infants do not apply to older children. The process is so difficult that only about half of all Medicaid-eligible children are actually enrolled. In addition, there are large differences in the benefits provided to children by the states (Rosenbaum 1988a: 44–45).

While the Medicaid expansions of the mid-1980s dealt with eligibility and enrollment issues, they did not address health care resource and delivery issues. This, of course, has always been a major characteristic of Medicaid policy.

Several factors have limited the number of providers available to care for low-income pregnant women in the U.S. First, there are the general problems of the geographical maldistribution of specialists and increasingly high rates of malpractice insurance for obstetrical practices. The latter has contributed to the decision of many gynecologist/obstetricians not to provide prenatal and childbirth services. In the U.S., the number of certified nurse midwives, an occupational group which has had great success in working with low-income as well as middle-income pregnant women, is extremely small (2,600) (IOM 1988: 66–69). "In some U.S. communities, particularly those with poorer populations and no teaching or public facilities, obstetrical care may be disappearing entirely" (ibid.: 69).

In areas where there are sufficient numbers of obstetricians, many of these physicians do not accept uninsured women or women with Medicaid as patients. Such women are viewed as requiring care that is more complicated and time-consuming than the care needed by privately insured women, and Medicaid fees are far below the usual charges paid to private specialists. Physicians also find Medicaid paperwork and delays in reimbursement burdensome. There is a belief among physicians that malpractice claims are substantially higher within the Medicaid population. For all of these reasons, many obstetricians (44 percent in a 1983 survey) will not treat women receiving Medicaid (ibid.: 66–69).

With limited access to the private sector, low-income pregnant women are likely to seek prenatal care at publicly funded clinics. The demand for such services has been increasing and the waiting time for prenatal appointments is long. An author of one study of public health and nonprofit hospital clinics is quoted by the Institute of Medicine: "A woman has to call for an appointment before she gets pregnant to get an appointment before the end of the first trimester" (ibid.: 66). Since half of all pregnancies in the U.S. are unplanned and probably a higher proportion of the pregnancies of women who use clinics are unplanned, this is clearly another barrier to access.

Such waiting time is related to the way in which Medicaid reimbursement policy has operated. Primary care clinics are reimbursed for services by only one-third of the states, and an additional one-third are reimbursed only for some of the services provided at such clinics. Outreach, health education, and counseling services provided by nonphysicians are not generally covered by Medicaid (Rosenbaum 1988a: 45). Community health centers, which were originally established to provide the type of care that experts now agree is necessary to reduce infant mortality and childhood illness in high-risk populations, have had their funding reduced since 1981.

Like their mothers, children whose health care is paid for by Medicaid are far less likely than are children in middle- and high-income families to be cared for by private practitioners. The same low fees, extensive paperwork, delays in processing, and retroactive denial of claims are viewed negatively by pediatricians, and their participation in the Medicaid program is limited. In 1983, the last year for which data was available, 53 percent of pediatricians nationwide either did not participate in Medicaid at all or accepted only a small number of Medicaid patients. The number of those not participating is believed to have increased since 1983.[3]

Clinics funded by the maternal and child health block grants serve only a small proportion of uninsured pregnant women and children. A survey of the agencies of all 50 states and the District of Columbia that were responsible

3. American Academy of Pediatrics, testimony on medical infant mortality initiatives before the Subcommittee on Health and the Environment, Committee on Energy and Commerce, U.S. House of Representatives, 8 February 1989.

for maternal and child health programs was conducted by the Children's Defense Fund during the summer of 1986. The purpose of the study was to determine whether those programs were meeting the needs of targeted populations. The survey respondents were state health officials. The study focused on services in four areas, outpatient prenatal care, inpatient maternity care, and outpatient and inpatient pediatric care. In all four areas, there was a lack of service relative to need (see Rosenbaum et al. 1988: 321–31).

Child health on the governmental agenda:
The framing of the issue

The way that an issue is defined or "framed" in public discourse is critical to the nature of activity on the issue, the type of groups that become involved, and the specific policies, if any, that are developed in response (Schattschneider 1960; Cobb and Elder 1972; Nelson 1984). The issues of reducing infant mortality and improving the health of children have been framed in such a way that makes them "valence-like" issues, issues that are consensual rather than conflictual for a large audience (Nelson 1984: 27–28).

Infant mortality and many childhood illnesses and disabilities have been defined as preventable, and thus as problems amenable to solution. A second major theme in the discussions of child health during the 1980s is that the provision of services in the present will save large health care costs later on. Third, investment in young children is said to be an investment in the U.S. economy, a theme related to concerns about the future of the American work force in a competitive international economy. Finally, child health is a valence-like issue because babies and young children, unlike other "disadvantaged groups," are viewed as innocents and morally blameless for their condition. In addition, since they are young, their lives can be changed and their problems are more "fixable" than those of adults. A number of governmental and non-governmental reports, as well as the statements of public officials, share this common framework as they discuss child health in the U.S. at the end of the 1980s.

Two of the influential "second-generation" government-sponsored studies on child health are a 1988 report of the Congressional Office of Technology Assessment (OTA) and a report by the National Commission to Prevent Infant Mortality issued in August 1988. The OTA study is an evaluation of the cost-effectiveness of various strategies to improve children's health, undertaken at the request of the Subcommittee on Health and the Environment of the House Energy and Commerce Committee and the Senate Labor and Human Resources Committee. The National Commission to Prevent Infant Mortality was created by Congress in 1986 in order to analyze public policies related to the health of women of reproductive age and infants. Its members included representatives of state government, members of Congress, Reagan administration officials, and health professionals with expertise in these areas. Maternal and child health issues have also recently been discussed by private sector organizations concerned with public policy. Two such discussions can be found in *Children in Need: Investment Strategies for the Educationally Disadvantaged*, issued in 1987 by the Committee for Economic Development, and *The Common Good, Social Welfare and the American Future*, published by the Ford Foundation in 1989. The Committee for Economic Development (CED) is a research and educational organization whose trustees include presidents and board chairmen of the largest American corporations. The content of its 1987 study is particularly interesting as a reflection of the views of some executives of large American corporations. While many corporate officials have expressed a strong interest in improving the public schools, the CED has included prenatal and child health services, nutrition counseling, and parenting education as part of its strategy for educational reform.

The consensus within the health policy community is that prenatal care improves the outcome of pregnancy, especially in populations at high risk. Demographically, high-risk pregnant women are likely to be young, black or Hispanic, unmarried, and poor (IOM 1988: 2–4). OTA reviewed 55 studies which examined the relationship between infant mortality and prenatal care and found that low birthweight and neonatal mortality can be reduced if mothers have early, "comprehensive" prenatal care (OTA 1988: 9).

The report of the Ford Foundation Project on Social Welfare and the American Future states, "Bringing a healthy baby into the world is something *we know how to do*, but too often in America we fail to do it" (Ford Foundation 1989: 12; emphasis added). The National Commission to Prevent Infant Mortality is explicit in framing infant mortality as a solvable problem in comparison to other policy issues: "Unlike other social problems, where cause and effect can blend together to obscure solutions, we know what we can do to halt the tragedy of infant mortality" (National Commission 1988: 10).

In addition to preventing the tragedy of the deaths of babies and young children, reducing infant mortality and improving children's health are viewed as ways of saving health care dollars. This argument gained much attention as the result of a study by the Institute of Medicine in 1985. That report linked low birthweight to infant mortality and disability, and argued that investing in prenatal care would save large sums of money that would not have to be spent on neonatal intensive care and other services for disabled children. Every dollar spent for prenatal care for high-risk women could save $3.38 in neonatal health costs (*National Journal* 1986a: 2257).

The theme that preventive interventions are cost-effective in terms of overall spending for health and social services was a major argument made for children's programs at the state level in the mid-1980s. Governors Michael N. Castle of Delaware, a Republican, and Martha Layne Collins of Kentucky, a Democrat, cochaired a National Governors Association "campaign" on children's programs. Castle states: "Investing in young children is like compound interest—the benefits, in reduced costs to society, accrue year after year." Governor Collins: "It's easier to build successful children than repair men and women. . . . Early childhood programs cost money and sometimes a lot of it. But crime costs more, overcrowded prisons cost more, welfare costs more, and undereducation costs more" (*National Journal* 1986b: 2849). This argument is still a central theme in all of the current policy discussions of maternal and child health services.

OTA analyzed the cost-effectiveness of a policy of Medicaid eligibility for all pregnant women with incomes below the federal poverty level and concluded that the cost of additional prenatal care would be more than paid for by saving the costs of hospitalization and other health care services associated with the birth of low-birthweight infants. OTA also calculated that childhood immunizations are cost-effective in these terms. There was not enough data to draw conclusions about the cost-effectiveness of other forms of well-child care (OTA 1988: 9–10, 13–14).

The National Commission to Prevent Infant Mortality uses OTA data to make the argument that providing health services to pregnant women and children will save money. Four hundred dollars spent on prenatal care saves between $14,000 and $30,000 in health costs for the care of a low-birthweight baby (a number which is an OTA estimate) and up to $400,000 for the care of a physically and/or mentally disabled person during his or her lifetime (National Commission 1988: 9).

In its report, *Children in Need*, the Committee for Economic Development includes a chart of "Cost-Effective Programs for Children." Included are WIC, Prenatal Care, Medicaid, and Childhood Immunization, as well as education and training programs. For each program, the cost benefit (e.g., "$1 spent on the Childhood Immunization program saves $10 in later medical costs") is stated. The Ford Foundation report says: "We can pay a little now to try to prevent blighted childhoods or we can pay a lot later for the consequences. In other words, money for decent prenatal care, or more than three times as much to deal with low-birthweight infants; several thousand dollars for a good preschool program to open the mind of a ghetto three-year-old, or tens of thousands of dollars to cope with a hardened teenage criminal" (Ford Foundation 1989: 11).

The argument that current spending for prenatal care can save money in the future was one of the major reasons for the popularity of infant mortality initiatives in the 101st Congress, a Congress in which children's issues in general had "high visibility" (*Congressional Quarterly* 1989b: 759). Supporters of such programs can be seen as both compassionate and financially prudent. According to former senator Lawton Chiles, the chairman of the National Commission to Prevent Infant Mortality, "It is not often that a person in public life gets to say 'I know how to save the lives of American children and save taxpayer money at the same time'" (ibid.: 760).

A separate economic argument made for supporting maternal and child health services (as well as education and nutrition programs) is that it is an investment in the future American work force. The title of the report of the Office of Technology Assessment is *Healthy Children: Investing in the Future*. The National Commission to Prevent Infant Mortality states that if our infant mortality rate were reduced to that of Japan's (the nation with the lowest rate in the world), the additional 20,000 children who survived each year would contribute $10 billion to the economy as workers (National Commission 1988: 10). The Ford Foundation report cites the dramatic decrease in the ratio of U.S. workers to retirees since 1950 and the need for a "highly skilled" labor force if the U.S. is to compete internationally (Ford Foundation 1989: 11-12). "We ought to invest in human capital with the same entrepreneurial spirit and concern for long-range payoffs that venture capitalists bring to investments in new enterprises" (ibid.: 46). In *Children in Need,* the Research and Policy Committee of the CED argues that the U.S. must educate the growing numbers of children in poverty if business is to find literate, skilled workers to do the intellectual tasks required by new levels of technology in both the manufacturing and service sectors of the economy. The CED report describes a "severe employment crisis" for business and a crisis in our political institutions if there is not widespread reform of our educational institutions. Part of the reform effort is "prevention through early intervention," including prenatal and postnatal care for high-risk mothers, well-child care, and parenting and nutrition education so that children will be able to learn in school (CED 1989: 4–5, 11).

Finally, the issue of health care for children fits comfortably into the American value system. Children are innocent in two different ways. First, they are malleable, "fixable" as adults may not be. They are, in a sense, a "new frontier" where we as a society can begin again and succeed in solving the social problems that frustrate us. Remember the statement of Governor Collins of Kentucky, quoted earlier: "It's easier to build successful children than repair men and women."

Second, children are innocent because they have not made a choice to do the things that many in the population would consider antisocial—i.e., taking illegal drugs, having children without being married, or receiving public assistance. Even among those with an individualistic view of the origins of social problems such as poverty and drug addiction, children can be seen as the victims of the actions of adults. According to a report done for the National Democratic Party in the fall of 1987, American voters do not resent government policies that help other people's *children*. There is far more support for social and economic programs that benefit children than for those that assist adults (*New York Times* 1987: 36). And focusing on children, as Marion Wright Edelman recognized when she founded the Children's Defense Fund in 1973, is probably the most comfortable way for Americans to deal with issues that are about race and class.

Beyond Medicaid expansion: Proposals for financing and restructuring health care delivery

The 1985 Institute of Medicine study on low birthweight was one of the key studies in mobilizing congressional opinion in support of the expansion of Medicaid eligibility for pregnant women and infants. Government-sponsored reports issued in the latter part of the 1980s make recommendations that deal with both the financing of child health services beyond the expansion of the Medicaid program and the restructuring of the health care delivery system. These proposals, as well as recommendations for short-term incremental change in the way that maternal and child health services are financed and delivered, will be reviewed next.

Universal maternal and child health services.   Both the Institute of Medicine and the National Commission to Prevent Infant Mortality are highly critical of maternal and infant health care services in the U.S. The Institute of Medicine's committee (IOM 1988: 36) to study outreach for prenatal care concluded that outreach was problematic in a system with so many financial, structural, and cultural barriers to care and calls upon our national leaders to "commit themselves openly and unequivocally to designing a new maternity system" (IOM 1988: 137). The system should be universal; provide services throughout pregnancy, childbirth, and the postpartum period; be accountable to a federal agency; use both physicians and certified midwives to provide care; and include a major program of public education and information. A commitment to family planning services must also be a central component in a universal maternity system, according to the IOM report, because women with unintended pregnancies are especially likely to delay prenatal care (ibid.: 139–40).

The National Commission to Prevent Infant Mortality also calls for "*universal access* to early maternity and pediatric care" and the elimination of "existing financial, administrative, logistical, geographical, educational, and social barriers to essential health services for pregnant women and infants" (National Commission 1988: 12; emphasis in original). It describes the successful post–World War II Japanese effort to reduce infant mortality, symbolized by the letter and handbook received by each Japanese woman when she registers her pregnancy (National Commission 1988: 9–10).

The commission takes the position that the private sector must take the "primary responsibility" for providing universal access to care. Prenatal and well-baby care should be a part of every employee's health benefit package, and coverage for these services should extend to spouses and dependents. Insurance pools should be established to assist small businesses in paying for employee health insurance; unincorporated businesses should be able to deduct the full cost of health insurance. These proposals are similar to those in legislation introduced in Congress by Senator Kennedy and Congressman Waxman, and will be discussed later in this chapter.

The commission also proposes a "permanent council" on children's health to conduct national education campaigns and coordinate public and private sector efforts, a contemporary Children's Bureau. It outlines an extensive political and educational campaign to make maternal and child health a major issue, involving the national media, business, labor, religious, and professional groups, and all levels of government (National Commission 1988: 22–23, 33–34).

The consensus that the U.S. must create a universal maternal and child health care system in order to reduce infant mortality is informed by studies of maternal and child health services in other nations. One such study is described in a paper by Dr. C. Arden Miller that was commissioned by the Institute of Medicine's committee to study outreach for prenatal care. That paper, "Prenatal Care Outreach: An International Perspective," will be summarized here.

Miller compared rates of low birthweight and infant mortality in ten European countries and the U.S., all countries with "mixed or pluralistic health care systems." He excluded from the study countries such as Finland and Sweden, where prenatal care is given exclusively by government personnel. In all countries except the United Kingdom, the rate of low birthweight was much lower than the overall U.S. rate as well as the rate for white babies in the U.S. Miller discussed several aspects of the comparative income and demographic characteristics of these European countries and the U.S. in relation to infant mortality rates. First, the average income in the United States is higher than in six of the countries with better infant mortality rates than the U.S. Second, while the gap between rich and poor is greater in the U.S. than in any other country except France, Denmark and Spain are close to the U.S. in inequality in distribution of income. Yet these countries have much lower rates of infant mortality than does the U.S. Third, the claim that the U.S. is more heterogeneous ethnically than Western Europe and therefore has significantly greater cultural barriers to overcome in delivering health care is belied by the substantial numbers of immigrant women of childbearing age now living in Western Europe. For instance, 44.5 percent of all children age 5 and under in Amsterdam in 1981 were born to non-Dutch families, primarily from Surinam and Morocco.

Miller used these data to argue that the high rates of infant mortality and low birthweight in the U.S. are a consequence of the absence of a maternal and child health care system here. Births to teenagers age 15–19 were three times higher in the U.S. than in Europe during the 1980s (within both the black and white populations), even though rates of abortion were lower in Western Europe than in the U.S. The age of onset of sexual activity does not vary across nations, but sex education and access to contraception are more widely available to European teenagers.

All of the nine European nations whose rates of low birthweight are lower than that of the U.S. have national standards for prenatal care, with organized community services at the local level and national financing and monitoring of these services. These countries are heterogeneous in terms of whether women use general practitioners, obstetricians, or midwives for prenatal and obstetrical care; in some countries women see more than one type of provider. In all of these countries, services are provided to all women, regardless of income, with minimal financial barriers to care. Incentives are provided for women to seek prenatal care, such as paid leave for prenatal classes or visits, transportation to services, early reservations for delivery, and children's allowances. Home visits are routinely made after delivery in every country but the U.S. There are much higher rates of participation in prenatal services in Western Europe than in the U.S.; fewer than 2 percent of women who give birth have had no prenatal care (Miller 1988: 210–27).

Social medicine proposals.   In addition to the need for a universal system of maternal and child health services, a second aspect of the consensus on child health is that infant mortality will only be reduced if prenatal and child health services address the social as well as the medical needs of high-risk mothers and children. "Our current health care system addresses infant mortality as a medical issue, rather than as a social problem with medical consequences" (National Commission 1988: 11).

In a 1988 book entitled *Within Our Reach: Breaking the Cycle of Disadvantage*, Lisbeth B. Schorr argues powerfully that only by employing what she calls (following the Robert Wood Johnson Foundation) a "transmedical" approach to health services will we be able to improve the health of low-income pregnant women and children. Such an approach provides a comprehensive, individualized, and integrated set of medical, nutritional, psychological, educational, and support services (Schorr 1988: 72–75).

Traditional prenatal care does not meet the needs of high-risk women. Low-income women may have histories of physical and sexual abuse and may be afraid of seeking gynecological care. Traditionally trained physicians are usually not successful in helping women with little education to understand the physical and psychological aspects of pregnancy, to stop using drugs, alcohol, or cigarettes, or to plan for parenting. Schorr quotes a nurse midwife working in the Southeast who says, "It can take an hour to establish rapport. If you're rushed, there's no communication. It takes time to enlist people—especially adolescents and very poor women—in their own care, and allow the discovery process to unfold" (ibid.: 71).

Schorr reviews specific prenatal care programs which taught women about pregnancy and parenting and were very successful in reducing infant mortality and low birthweight. One was a program run by Johns Hopkins University Hospital from a Baltimore storefront. The patients in the program were primarily black, low-income, unmarried teenagers, all seventeen or younger. The program was small, so that the staff—including a community outreach worker who made home visits, a social worker, a health educator, an obstetrical nurse, and an obstetrician—could have a personal relationship with each patient. Health education sessions were held before each clinical visit. An evaluation of the program between 1979 and 1981 compared patient outcomes in the storefront group with those of a matched group of teenagers receiving basic prenatal and obstetrical care at other Johns Hopkins programs. The rate of low birthweight was 60 percent greater in the control group than in the storefront program.

In a South Carolina program called "Resource Mothers" (funded by the Robert Wood Johnson Foundation), community women in a poor rural area were trained to teach pregnant teenagers about nutrition, pregnancy, childbirth, and parenting. These older women would meet each girl at least once a month, help them to apply for social service benefits, and supply information and support. Again, in comparison to a control group, these teenagers gave birth to far fewer low-birthweight infants and had healthier babies up to age 1 (ibid.: 77–83).

Schorr argues that the same integrated social, educational, and medical approach is necessary to provide adequate health services to high-risk children, most of whom are at high risk because of their social and physical environment. She reviews health programs for children that used a transmedical approach, in which transportation, nutrition, outreach services, and parenting education were available and in which long-term relationships developed between families and staff (ibid.: 85–110). She quotes Dr. Aaron Shirley, who has worked at community health centers in poor black areas of Mississippi for more than twenty years: "Our outreach workers are not frills, our attempts to eliminate barriers and to maintain a friendly atmosphere are not trivial, the broad range of services we offer is not a luxury. For many of the families we see, all these are an absolute necessity" (ibid.: 97). Schorr emphasizes the importance of restructuring financing so that counseling, health education, and other social and educational services have a stable, ongoing source of funding (ibid.: 122).

The National Commission to Prevent Infant Mortality makes several recommendations which would be part of a "transmedical" or "social medicine" approach to maternal and child health care. It proposes nutrition programs, greater numbers of programs to reduce substance abuse among women of reproductive age, and education programs to prevent unintended pregnancies. It suggests training "indigenous community outreach workers" to provide social support services and a "home visitors" program for pregnant women and infants (National Commission 1988: 29–30). In July 1989, the National Commission issued a booklet entitled "Home Visiting: Opening Doors for America's Pregnant Women and Children," with the printed pages in the shape of a house. It describes the history of home visiting, contemporary home visiting in England and Denmark, and specific demonstration programs in the U.S. The booklet argues that home visiting is a cost-effective method for reducing low birthweight as well as child neglect and abuse, and for promoting the growth and development of children by improving parenting and nurturing skills, reducing smoking and drug and alcohol abuse, increasing the use of prenatal and well-child care, and reducing the use of inappropriate emergency room visits. More broadly, it states that high-technology, narrowly medical approaches to maternal and child health are very limited in their effectiveness. Rather, it is social support services that are critical if infant mortality is to be further reduced in the U.S. (National Commission 1989: 1).

The Office of Technology Assessment is somewhat more cautious about home visitor programs because one-to-one counseling and support services are costly. It suggests that Congress fund experimental home visitor programs for women and families at risk for low-birthweight babies and child maltreatment (OTA 1988: 23–24).

One of the major themes of the Institute of Medicine's study on prenatal care is that both in creating a new system of maternal and infant health services and in short-term efforts to improve care, the social needs of women should be of central concern. These needs include the opportunity to have an ongoing relationship with health care providers sensitive to their culture and language, time to talk about unfamiliar procedures, convenient appointment times and locations, child care, and home visiting (IOM 1988: 14–15, 146–47).

Proposals for incremental reform.   Although the Institute of Medicine report calls for the restructuring of maternal and child health care in the U.S., it also proposes some incremental steps to make prenatal care more accessible in the short run. Like the National Commission to Prevent Infant Mortality, the Institute of Medicine calls for an expansion of maternity services provided by private insurance (ibid.: 143). In addition to providing greater financial access to care through the private sector, there is agreement on other short-term means of increasing access to care. These include further Medicaid expansion, reforms in the Medicaid application process, and increasing the number of physicians and institutions serving low-income women and children.

The Institute of Medicine recommends that the Medicaid eligibility level for pregnant women be increased to 185 percent of the poverty level and then further expanded (ibid.: 142); the National Commission to Prevent Infant Mortality proposes that all pregnant women and infants with family incomes at or below 200 percent of the poverty level be eligible for Medicaid (National Commission 1988: 18). The position of the American Academy of Pediatrics is that Medicaid should be provided to children up to age 21 whose family incomes are at or below the poverty level.[4]

There is agreement that complicated application forms, long waiting times between application and notification of eligibility, asset tests, and other bureaucratic obstacles are barriers to care and should be eliminated (IOM 1988: 71–73; National Commission 1988: 18, 21; OTA 1988: 20, 87). There is also a consensus that expanding eligibility for Medicaid without assuming that there are adequate services available is counterproductive. The National Commission and the Institute of Medicine recommend that Medicaid reimbursement rates be raised and administrative requirements be simplified in order to increase provider participation in Medicaid. The OTA suggests that the number of EPSDT-required visits be reduced and the additional money be used to pay higher fees for EPSDT screening and immunization (National Commission 1988: 21; IOM 1988: 144; OTA 1988: 22–23). There is also agreement that the malpractice "crisis" in obstetrics needs to be addressed and funding for existing federal programs that provide services to pregnant women and children should be expanded (National Commission 1988: 20, 21; IOM 1988: 141, 144; OTA 1988: 25).

A bipartisan group of legislators supported Medicaid expansion in the 101st Congress. In addition to enlarging the Medicaid-eligible population, legislative provisions passed in 1989 address the Medicaid application process, increasing physician participation in the Medicaid program, the coordination of federal programs serving pregnant women and children, and home visiting as a federally funded service. I will briefly review these legislative efforts to improve child health and conclude with some speculations on the political viability of the current "consensus" on child health issues.

Child health legislation for fiscal years 1990 and 1991

Competition to support Medicaid expansion.   As a presidential candidate, George Bush supported federally mandated Medicaid eligibility for all children living in families with incomes below the poverty level and "measures to phase in affordable coverage for pregnant women and infants up to 185 percent of poverty" through employer-based coverage and Medicaid buy-ins. His campaign memo on child health fits clearly within the bipartisan consensus that developed during the 1980s. High infant mortality rates can be reduced by decreasing the incidence of teenage pregnancy and by providing

---

4. American Academy of Pediatrics, Medicaid policy statement, January 1986.

universal access to prenatal care, health education, and nutrition for pregnant women. The argument is also made that reducing the proportion of low-birthweight babies is cost-effective for the health care system.[5] Since his election, the president and congressional health activists have competed for sponsorship of child health legislation (*Congressional Quarterly* 1989e: 1552).

Bush proposed in his fiscal year 1990 budget that Medicaid coverage be mandated for pregnant women and infants with family incomes at or below 130 percent of the poverty level. In February 1989, Congressman Henry A. Waxman and Senator Bill Bradley introduced the Medicaid Child Health Amendments of 1989 into the House and Senate. These bills would require states to expand Medicaid eligibility to all pregnant women and infants in families with incomes up to 185 percent of the federal poverty level ($17,900 for a family of three) by 1993 and phase in Medicaid coverage for children up to age 18 living in families with incomes below the poverty level. At a press conference to announce the introduction of the bill, Waxman and Bradley were joined by Congressmen Henry J. Hyde and Mickey Leland, ideological opposites on most issues of social policy (*Congressional Quarterly* 1989a: 221; Waxman 1989: 1217).

In March 1989, Congressman George Miller, chair of the House Select Committee on Children and Youth, and Congressman Waxman introduced the Child Health and Security Act. This legislation would authorize expansions of Medicaid eligibility for pregnant women, infants, and children up to 200 percent of the poverty level, expand eligibility for the WIC program, and increase funds for an Infant Mortality Initiative at Community and Migrant Health Centers, the Head Start programs, and child health immunization programs. Home visiting for prenatal and postpartum visits would be mandated services under Medicaid. Congressman Miller discussed this comprehensive legislation as a cost-effective investment in the nation's future (*Congressional Record* 1989: E936).

Legislation expanding Medicaid eligibility for pregnant women, infants, and children passed the House on 5 October 1989. The eligibility levels approved were those in the Waxman-Bradley bill. In addition, states were not to be allowed to consider family assets in determining Medicaid eligibility for pregnant women and infants. States were also to be required to conduct the Medicaid application process for pregnant women, infants, and children at hospitals, clinics, and other locations that are not welfare offices, and to notify all Medicaid-eligible women and children under age 5 that they are eligible for the WIC program.[6]

---

5. "Invest in Our Children," statement from the 1988 Bush-Quayle campaign, October 1988.

6. Summary of Medicaid budget reconciliation provisions as reported by the Committee on Energy and Commerce, U.S. House of Representatives, 13 July 1989.

The Senate Finance Committee approved Medicaid expansions which were not as large as those approved by the House. Eligibility was to be mandated for pregnant women and children to age 6 in families with incomes at or below 133 percent of the federal poverty level. States could provide Medicaid to all children up to age 19 in families with incomes at or below the poverty level (*Congressional Quarterly* 1989h: 2642).

Legislation to improve health care delivery.   The Medicaid legislation passed as part of the House reconciliation bill for fiscal year 1990 also addressed several health care delivery issues. Beginning 1 July 1990, states were to submit information annually to the secretary of the Department of Health and Human Services (DHHS) on Medicaid rates for obstetrical and pediatric services. The secretary was to decide whether these levels of reimbursement would "assure a reasonable level of provider participation in the program."[7] The Subcommittee on Health and the Environment would have funded state demonstration programs to increase participation in Medicaid by pediatricians and obstetricians,[8] but this provision was not passed by the full committee.

The Medicaid legislation passed by the House also allowed states to pay for home visits to high-risk pregnant women and children if prescribed by a doctor. States were also required to reimburse federally funded community health centers for ambulatory services provided to pregnant women and children "on a reasonable cost basis."[9]

Legislation aimed at improving the delivery of prenatal and infant care services by eliminating some of the current "geographic, administrative, cultural, logistical and educational" barriers to care[10] was introduced into both houses of Congress in April 1989 by four members of the National Commission to Prevent Infant Mortality. The Healthy Birth Act of 1989 would have added $100 million to the fiscal year 1990 Maternal and Child Health Services Block Grant to be used for state-sponsored demonstration programs of up to five years. These programs would include home visits to pregnant women and infants, centers where pregnant women and mothers could apply for all state and federal programs for which they are eligible ("one-stop shopping"), and statewide toll-free hot lines that could make referrals for maternal and child health services. The federal government would be required to distribute a national maternal and child health handbook (with information on pregnancy and parenting), to develop a simplified, combined application for Medicaid,

---

7. See footnote 6.
8. Summary of the Medicaid Reconciliation Provisions as approved by the Subcommittee on Health and the Environment, 29 June 1989.
9. See footnote 6.
10. The National Commission to Prevent Infant Mortality, "The Healthy Birth Act of 1989," p. 1.

WIC, and other federal programs, and to establish a national maternal and child health services hot line (*Congressional Quarterly* 1989b: 759–60).

The House approved provisions for home visiting and the development of a coordinated application process for federal maternal and child health programs as part of the legislation reauthorizing the Maternal and Child Health Services Block Grant for fiscal year 1990, but did not include funding for a national telephone hot line or a maternal and child handbook. The Senate Finance Committee authorized $711 million for the Maternal and Child Health Services Block Grant, $50 million more than authorized by the full House, but was less expansive than the House in approving outreach efforts for pregnant women and infants. The Senate Finance Committee provided funding for fewer demonstration projects involving home visiting than did the House and required only that each state that received funding through the Maternal and Child Health Services Block Grant develop a plan to determine how pregnant women and children could apply for a variety of federal health, nutrition, and social service programs at one location. The House bill required that the secretary of DHHS develop a model application form for such a "one-stop shopping" process of applying for federal programs. However, the Senate Appropriations Committee approved $1 million for the development of a maternal and child health handbook in the fiscal year 1990 budget bill (*Congressional Quarterly* 1989h: 2462).[11]

The fiscal year 1990 reconciliation bill was passed on 22 November 1989, after several weeks of deadlock over the capital gains tax and general deficit reduction issues. It requires that states provide Medicaid to all pregnant women, infants, and children up to age 6 in families with incomes up to 133 percent of the poverty level beginning on 1 April 1990 (*Congressional Quarterly* 1989i: 3447). The Children's Defense Fund estimates that one million children between the ages of 1 and 6 will gain Medicaid coverage as a result of this legislation (Children's Defense Fund 1990: 6). The Omnibus Reconciliation Act of 1989 also mandates that states reimburse obstetrical and pediatric providers at levels high enough to give Medicaid patients access to care equal to the "general population" of their area (states must submit these rates to the federal government annually), that states reimburse all federally qualified community health centers for services under the Medicaid program at "100 percent of their reasonable costs" and that the services of pediatric and family nurse practitioners be reimbursed by state Medicaid programs, whether or not the nurse practitioners are affiliated with a physician.

The 1989 legislation makes significant changes in the EPSDT program for Medicaid-eligible children. States are now required to provide screening ex-

---

11. Telephone interviews with a professional staff member of the National Commission to Prevent Infant Mortality, 25 September and 1 November 1989. Also see footnote 6.

aminations for medical, vision, dental, and hearing problems at specific intervals and between these intervals when a new problem (or a worsening condition) appears to exist. Health education of children and advice to parents have been added as required parts of the EPSDT screening examination. States are now mandated to provide any federally funded Medicaid service necessary to treat a condition found during a screening examination, even if the service is not part of that state's Medicaid program. Federal rules about provider participation are clarified so that a larger pool of providers will be qualified to do EPSDT screening exams. New annual state EPSDT reporting requirements and federal program goals are also mandated (ibid.: 17–24).

The authorization level for the Maternal and Child Health Services Block Grant was raised from $561 million to $686 million (*Congressional Quarterly* 1989i: 3447–48), but the actual fiscal year 1990 appropriation for maternal and child health was only $554 million because of reductions made in all programs in order to meet the requirements of the Gramm-Rudman budget legislation. This was the same level of program funding as in FY 1989.

The fiscal year 1990 reconciliation bill also contains a provision that when the funding of the Maternal and Child Health Services Block Grant reaches $600 million, states will be required to use a certain proportion of the funds to establish demonstration programs which involve home visiting, to develop coordinated applications for federal maternal and child health, nutrition, and social service programs, and to support several other innovations in the delivery of care.[12]

The fiscal year 1991 budget reconciliation bill (HR 5835), which was passed during the last week of October 1990, expands Medicaid eligibility for children from age 6 through age 18. States are required to phase in this broadened coverage for children who live in families with incomes at or below the poverty level by the year 2002 (*Washington Post* 1990: A4). This is essentially the Waxman-Bradley bill proposed in 1989.

The Budget Reconciliation Act of 1990 also mandates that pregnant women be covered by Medicaid throughout their pregnancy and for 60 days after delivery, that infants be covered until their first birthday without recertifying family income, that states provide shortened Medicaid applications at hospitals, community health centers and other places outside of welfare offices. It also establishes minimum qualifications for physicians participating in the Medicaid program (Children's Defense Fund Memorandum 1990a: 1–3).

The appropriation for the Maternal and Child Health Services Block grant for fiscal year 1991 is $587.3 million (Children's Defense Fund Memorandum 1990b), an increase of 6 percent over the 1990 level, not high enough to trigger state-sponsored demonstration programs which involve transmedical services.

---

12. Telephone interview with a professional staff member of the National Commission to Prevent Infant Mortality, 16 February 1990.

The secretary of DHHS is also required to develop and distribute a maternal and child handbook targeted at "high-risk" families and to develop a model "one-stop shopping" application within a year (ibid.: 3448). However, states are not required to adopt this model application.[13] States are required to assess maternal and child health needs every five years and must establish toll-free telephone numbers to inform families about the availability of health services (ibid.: 3448).

By requiring that independent nurse practitioners and community health centers be included as Medicaid providers in all states and that Medicaid rates for obstetrical and pediatric services be increased, and that physicians who participate in the Medicaid program meet minimum qualifications, the 1990 and 1991 legislation makes it more likely that low-income women and children will have access to ongoing, appropriate primary health care services.[14] The changes in the EPSDT program also have the potential to greatly improve the comprehensiveness of service delivery to Medicaid-eligible children. Several provisions of the fiscal year 1990 reconciliation bill also begin to deal with the critical problems of lack of information about where to seek care and the bureaucratic barriers in the application process. However, the reconciliation legislation does not address the fundamental problem of the fragmentation and underfunding of child health services. And, other than providing for future demonstration projects that include home visiting and mandating that states must provide all Medicaid services necessary to treat a condition discovered during an EPSDT exam, it does not specifically fund transmedical services. The consensus on child health may not be broad enough or the commitment to the issue deep enough to overcome current obstacles to social welfare spending in general.

Child health policy and health care politics: Speculation on the future

The reduction of a high national infant mortality rate and the improvement of access to care for poor women and children became major issues on the health policy agenda during the 1980s. The response of Congress has been incremental reform, in the form of expansions of Medicaid eligibility. While a policy community concerned with the health of children discusses universal access and outreach programs such as those found in other industrial democracies, congressional initiatives in this direction have thus far been limited to authorizing funding for home visiting and appropriating money for the development of a national maternal and child health handbook.

---

13. See footnote 12.
14. In 1988, two-thirds of the six million people receiving health care at community health centers were women of reproductive age and children (Children's Defense Fund 1990: 10).

The future of maternal and child health policy is not clear. On the one hand, there are public officials and private groups actively working to move policy toward greater access to care; on the other, opposition to further government mandates on child health has already emerged.

The National Commission to Prevent Infant Mortality has argued that a universal maternal and child health system should be based on the expansion of private sector employee health insurance plans. At the state level, child health advocacy organizations such as the CDF and chapters of the American Academy of Pediatrics (AAP) have been working to enact legislation mandating preventive child health care—"child health supervision services"— as a part of all health insurance plans. As of the summer of 1989, six states required such coverage, and legislation mandating that health insurance plans provide preventive child health services had been introduced into the state legislatures of ten other states. State AAP chapters have also worked for state legislation requiring employers to provide health insurance to their employees, for the expansion of Medicaid eligibility, for the improvement of Medicaid reimbursement levels for physicians, and for the creation of high-risk pools at the state level which would include benefits for disabled children. AAP officials and staff view these activities as groundwork for a universal child health plan at the federal level (American Academy of Pediatrics 1989).

The AAP's "highest priority" for the next several years is to provide access to health services, including preventive care, to all pregnant women and all children up to age 21 (AAP News 1989: 1). Universality would be achieved through the existing employment-based system of health insurance. The federal government would require employers to provide health insurance to their employees and states would administer a public fund (financed by a tax on employers who did not provide a minimum benefits package to their employees) to pay for health services for the unemployed (ibid.: 8).

Recent efforts by Senator Edward M. Kennedy and Congressman Henry A. Waxman to enact legislation mandating that all employers provide a minimum health insurance plan has met with opposition from small business, the health insurance industry, and the Bush administration. The Chamber of Commerce and the National Federation of Independent Business oppose the Kennedy-Waxman legislation even though it contains several "sweeteners" to small business, such as government subsidies and postponement of compliance. No action was taken on the House bill during the 100th Congress legislative session. The Senate Labor and Human Resources Committee approved the bill, but it was not enacted in the full Senate (*Congressional Quarterly* 1989c: 826–27; *New York Times* 1989: E4). A similar bill was approved by Labor and Human Resources in July 1989, but its future is uncertain since the small business community and the Bush administration continue to oppose it (*Congressional Quarterly* 1989f: 1784).

In addition to the opposition to mandating the expansion of health insurance in the private sector, opposition to further expansion of Medicaid eligibility via federal mandates has developed and raises questions about whether this can continue to be a viable incremental strategy. The opposition has come from the National Governors Association (NGA), a group which lobbied for the original expansions of Medicaid eligibility. At its annual meeting in August 1989, the NGA passed a resolution asking Congress and the president not to enact further Medicaid mandates for a two-year period. The governors cited the high cost of these mandates to their states as the reason for their opposition. They also called for an examination of broader reform (*Congressional Quarterly* 1989g: 2121–23).

The provisions of the Budget Reconciliation Act of 1990 requiring phased-in Medicaid coverage for all poor children up to age 19 were passed in spite of opposition from the National Governors' Association and the Bush administration. The coalition supporting this Medicaid expansion included not only children's advocacy groups, pediatricians, and children's hospitals but also the American Medical Association, the American Hospital Association, the Blue Cross and Blue Shield Association, the Health Insurance Association of America (HIAA), the U.S. Chamber of Commerce, and the National Association of Manufacturers. The health insurers, business groups, and institutional providers who were members of this coalition viewed the expansion of Medicaid as a way to reduce the amount of uncompensated health care by decreasing the number of uninsured children (*New York Times* 1990: 24). Businesses pay for the uninsured when provider costs are shifted to them through higher premiums charged for insured workers. The president of the HIAA gave another reason for the support of the commercial health insurance industry: reducing the numbers of the uninsured would reduce the likelihood of a consensus developing on the need for a national health insurance program (ibid.).

While the expansion of Medicaid may be seen as a way to forestall pressure for a major restructuring of health care financing, it is also a means by which businesses can socialize their costs. While businesses would pay for their workers' insurance under a mandated employer-based plan, the expansion of Medicaid, paid for from general tax revenues, spreads the cost among all taxpayers.

Broader reform in the financing of child health services was proposed by Congressman Pete Stark, chairman of the Subcommittee on Health of the House Ways and Means Committee, when he introduced a bill (H.R. 4280) in March 1990, amending the Social Security Act to provide comprehensive health insurance to all pregnant women and to children up to age 23. The "Medicare program" for children would be financed by a payroll tax (H.R. 4280). The bill was introduced as a "discussion piece," to put the issue of comprehensive health insurance for mothers and children on the congressional agenda. It will be reintroduced early in the 102d Congress, but there are no plans to push for enactment in 1991.[15]

Moving beyond the agenda-building phase of the policy process would raise issues of the cost of such a program within the context of the politics of the budget deficit,[16] as well as ideological concerns about state expansion, which are triggered whenever universality is proposed in American social welfare policy.

What possible constituencies can child health advocacy groups and pediatricians enlist on behalf of greater access? And what other cleavages and/or conflicts would emerge if there were further movement toward universality?

One such constituency is business. In an article in *The Atlantic* entitled "Kids as Capital," Jonathan Rauch reviews discussions about children's issues which are said to be occurring in corporate boardrooms and among conservative as well as liberal policy analysts. He reiterates the development of the widespread consensus that a future labor force of adults who grew up in poverty will not be able to support the baby boom generation in its retirement. Business is now interested in children because this has become a matter of "self-interest." These concerns of corporate America, Rauch suggests, may be the basis of a new set of family-oriented policies that will "socialize" child rearing in order to guarantee a healthy, skilled "national family" (Rauch 1989: 56–61). Research is needed to assess the extent to which this kind of thinking is found within business elites as represented by the CED discussed earlier and to evaluate the degree of commitment to such a social policy agenda.

Another potential constituency is a mobilized public. The National Commission to Prevent Infant Mortality in its role as policy entrepreneur on the issue of infant mortality called for the media to educate the public on maternal and child health issues. Public television responded with a documentary on child health in the spring of 1989. In August 1989, *Parenting*, a magazine aimed at the college-educated population with young children, included an article on prenatal care entitled "The Preventable Tragedy." It presents the stories of several women who could not get access to prenatal care, even though they sought it assiduously. Interspersed with these stories of tragedy and near tragedy were data on infant death rates, low birthweight, access to

---

15. Telephone interview with staff member of House Ways and Means Committee, 31 January 1991.

16. The expansions of Medicaid eligibility and other cost-generating provisions in the Medicaid and Medicare legislation for fiscal year 1991 are supposed to be offset by a number of cost-cutting provisions, such as requiring pharmaceutical companies to discount prescription drugs for Medicaid patients and requiring states to pay for the premiums of employed workers whose family members might otherwise be eligible for Medicaid (Children's Defense Fund Memorandum 1990: 2).

care, and a discussion of all of the structural conditions related to infant mortality in the U.S.: high malpractice insurance, low Medicaid rates, overcrowded public clinics, etc. Most interestingly, the article includes a "Parent Action Plan," urging readers to write to state and national legislators and to lobby on this issue. In September 1990, the *New York Times Magazine* published an article entitled "Why Is America Failing Its Children?" by T. Berry Brazelton, a nationally known pediatrician and a member of the National Commission on Children. Brazelton discussed the work of the commission, a group established in 1989, which will issue its report in the spring of 1991. In October 1990, *Time* magazine's cover story provided a comprehensive assessment of American children's health, educational, and social needs and the limited public programs designed to meet those needs. Direct comparisons were made with the family policies of several European nations (Gibbs 1990: 42–46). Many other popular magazines and newspapers have recently included stories on U.S. infant mortality and child health. The diffusion of research on child abuse from scientific and professional journals to the national media was an important factor in making child abuse a salient issue to the public (Nelson 1984: 57–61). A similar process is occurring with broader maternal and child health issues. This could help create an "interested public" on child health issues which, in turn, would increase the number of members of Congress who would support policy change. Indeed, when people were asked by the Roper Organization, Inc., whether "investment" in children's health should be increased in spite of the budget deficit, 71 percent said yes (*National Journal* 1990: 2093). If the article in *Parenting* is the beginning of a similar process on broader maternal and child health issues, it could help create an "interested public." Certainly the demonstration of widespread concern on this issue by citizens who vote will enlarge the number of members of Congress who support policy change.

Even if a commitment from corporate elites emerged and a large number of citizens were mobilized, fundamental policy change is problematic because of the nature of our political institutions. The system of shared powers and decentralized legislatures without significant party discipline allows narrow opposition groups to prevent policy change. The existence of such groups with regard to further Medicaid expansion and the broadening of employment-based health insurance has already been discussed. Lessons from the history of child health policy in the U.S. suggest that if broader financing plans proceed, physicians' groups might oppose the widespread use of less expensive health professionals (such as certified nurse midwives) to deliver care.

The American Academy of Pediatrics is the most liberal of physician professional associations and has a history of advocacy for increasing access to child health services. Yet pediatricians at the local level were not happy when other health professionals were to provide publicly supported services in the EPSDT program. In California, Arkansas, and some other states, pediatricians opposed the use of public health nurses and nurse practitioners to do EPSDT screening (Goggin 1987: 87, 155).

In most states, screening was done by public clinics and referrals for treatment made to the patients' "usual source of care." This separation of screening and treatment was a result of state responsiveness to the concerns of private practitioners, particularly pediatricians. In Texas, EPSDT screening clinics, staffed by nurses, were not even allowed to treat minor conditions such as scabies (body lice), because this would have been "unacceptable" to the Texas Medical Association (Foltz 1982: 108, 113). The consequence of the separation of screening and treatment was that the EPSDT program did not create an integrated system of preventive and treatment services for Medicaid eligible children (Foltz 1982: 167–68). In many states, screening sites continue to be separate from other sources of care (OTA 1988: 22–23).

Another potential arena of conflict is the provision of primary care to teenagers and preteenagers in school-based health clinics. Services provided at such clinics are believed to have reduced the rate of teenage pregnancy in the communities in which they operate. They are the only source of primary health care for many low-income adolescents. Although fewer than 25 percent of all clinic visits at the approximately 160 school health clinics in the U.S. are for any type of reproductive health services, such clinics are opposed by anti-abortion groups, Christian fundamentalists, and the Catholic church. In Alexandria, Virginia, the mayor's support for a citywide health clinic for adolescents became a major issue in his 1988 election campaign (McCormick 1989: 56–61).

These potential conflicts over professional turf and social values will become significant if broader programs for prenatal care and children's health services are formulated and implemented. At the beginning of the 1990s, the prospect of further action toward universal access to maternal and child health care appears to recede in the face of tremendous concern with the U.S. budget deficit.

Conclusion

The future of U.S. child health policy depends on the large question of how policymakers resolve the tension between concern with federal budget deficits and concern with our "mounting social deficit" (Ford Foundation 1989: 2). American economic, fiscal, and social policies stand together here at a fundamental watershed. Incremental policy change on behalf of children has been popular because children's health problems appear to be solvable in a way that our other social crises do not. Although this focus on children has been tactically correct in terms of achieving some policy change, it obscures the complicated web of economic and social forces that produce low-birthweight babies and sick and disabled children.

Children live in families and in communities. To become a society that produces healthy infants and children, we must deal with adult employment and family income, education, drug use, and housing issues. A universal prenatal and primary health care system providing transmedical services to pregnant women and children must be part of a comprehensive set of employment, wage, child care, and housing policies that support both the adults and children in families.

References

AAP News. 1989. Congressional Staff, Health Experts Discuss Access Laws. February, pp. 1, 8.

American Academy of Pediatrics. 1989. Access to Care: The Role of State Chapters. CHIRP Victories in Minnesota and Connecticut. *Child Health Financing Report*, Spring/Summer, pp. 1, 3.

Black, J. E. 1988. The Sentimental Marketplace: Who Controls Child Health Care? In *Money, Power and Health Care*, ed. E. Melhado, W. Feinberg, and H. M. Schwartz. Ann Arbor, MI: Health Administration Press.

Brazelton, T. B. 1990. Why Is America Failing Its Children? *New York Times Magazine*, 9 September, pp. 40–42, 50, 90.

Children's Defense Fund. 1989. *The Health of America's Children: Maternal and Child Health Data Book*. Washington, DC: Children's Defense Fund.

———. 1990. *Report on 1989 Maternal and Child Health Federal Legislation*. Washington, DC: Children's Defense Fund.

Children's Defense Fund Memorandum. 1990a. Selected Medicaid Reforms in the Budget Reconciliation Act of 1990. 2 November, pp. 1–3.

Children's Defense Fund Memorandum, 1990b. Appropriations for Key Maternal and Child Health Programs. 25 October.

Cobb, R. W., and c. D. Elder. 1972. *Participation in American Politics: The Dynamics of Agenda-Building*. Baltimore, MD: Johns Hopkins University Press.

Committee for Economic Development. 1987. *Children in Need: Investment Strategies for the Educationally Disadvantaged*. New York: Committee for Economic Development.

Congressional Quarterly Weekly Report. 1989a. Broad Plans to Revise Health Insurance Offered. 4 February, p. 221.

———. 1989b. Drop in U.S. Infant Mortality Goal of New Legislation. 8 April, pp. 759–60.

———. 1989c. Kennedy, Waxman Introduce Insurance-for-All Proposal. 15 April, pp. 826–27.

———. 1989d. Reconciliation Dominates Policy-Making Process. 29 April, pp. 964–68.

———. 1989e. Medicaid Plan Would Reach 2 Million More Children. 24 June, p. 1552.

———. 1989f. Mandated-Benefits Legislation OK'd by Senate Committee. 15 July, p. 1784.

————. 1989g. Governors' Medicaid Protests Likely to Be Swept Aside. 12 August, pp. 2121–23.

————. 1989h. Medicare Payments to Doctors Revised by Senate Finance. 7 October, pp. 2641–42.

————. 1989i. Deficit-Reduction Bill Offers $14.7 Billion in Cuts. 16 December, pp. 3442–53.

Congressional Record. 1989. 101st Cong., 1st sess. 22 March.

Davis, K., and C. Schoen. 1978. *Health and the War on Poverty.* Washington, DC: Brookings Institution.

Foltz, A. M. 1982. *An Ounce of Prevention: Child Health Politics Under Medicaid.* Cambridge, MA: MIT Press.

Ford Foundation Project on Social Welfare and the American Future. 1989. *The Common Good, Social Welfare and the American Future.* New York: Ford Foundation.

Geiger, H. J. 1984. Community Health Centers: Health Care as an Instrument of Social Change. In *Reforming Medicine: Lessons of the Last Quarter Century*, ed. V. W. Sidel and R. Sidel. New York: Pantheon Books.

Gibbs, N. 1990. Shameful Bequests to the Next Generation. *Time*, 8 October, pp. 42–46.

Goggin, M. L. 1987. *Policy Design and the Politics of Implementation: The Case of Child Health Care in the American States.* Knoxville: University of Tennessee Press.

Halpern, S. A. 1988. *American Pediatrics: The Social Dynamics of Professionalism, 1880–1980.* Berkeley: University of California Press.

Institute of Medicine, ed. 1988. *Prenatal Care: Reaching Mothers, Reaching Infants.* Washington, DC: National Academy Press.

Kimmich, M. H. 1985. *America's Children: Who Cares?* Washington, DC: The Urban Institute Press.

Knowles, J. H. 1977. The Responsibility of the Individual. *Daedalus* 106 (1): 57–80.

Marieskind, H. I. 1980. *Women in the Health System: Patients, Providers, and Programs.* St. Louis, MO: C. V. Mosby.

McCormick, K. 1989. Bringing Health Care to the Kids. *Governing*, pp. 56–61.

Miller, C. A. 1988. Prenatal Care Outreach: An International Perspective. In *Prenatal Care: Reaching Mothers, Reaching Infants*, ed. Institute of Medicine. Washington, DC: National Academy Press.

National Commission to Prevent Infant Mortality. 1988. *Death Before Life: The Tragedy of Infant Mortality.* Washington, DC: National Commission to Prevent Infant Mortality.

————. 1989. *Home Visiting: Opening Doors for America's Pregnant Women and Children.* Washington, DC: National Commission to Prevent Infant Mortality.

National Journal. 1986a. Concern About Children. 20 September, pp. 2255–58.

————. 1986b. Children's Agenda Making Headway in States. 22 November, p. 2849.

————. 1988. Not Just Kids' Stuff. 19 November, pp. 2934–39.

————. 1989. Watch Out for Waxman. 11 March, pp. 577–81.

————. 1990. Opinion Outlook. 1 September, p. 2093.

Nelson, B. J. 1984. *Making an Issue of Child Abuse*. Chicago: University of Chicago Press.

New York Times. 1983. Now, a Select Committee for Families. 23 February, p. A18.

———. 1987. Children Emerge as Issue for Democrats. 27 September, p. 36.

———. 1989. Sudden Support for National Health Care. 24 September, p. E4.

———. 1990. Deficit or No Deficit, Unlikely Allies Bring about Expansion in Medicaid. 4 November, p. 24.

Oberg, C. N., and C. L. Polich. 1988. Medicaid: Entering the Third Decade. *Health Affairs* 7 (4): 83–96.

Parenting. 1989. The Preventable Tragedy. August, pp. 69–77.

Rauch, J. 1989. Kids as Capital. *The Atlantic*, August, pp. 56–61.

Rinehart, S. T. 1987. Maternal Health Care Policy: Britain and the United States. *Comparative Politics* 19 (2): 193–211.

Rosenbaum, S. 1988a. *Lives in the Balance*. Manuscript in progress.

———. 1988b. Update on Maternal and Child Health Developments: Memorandum to State Primary Care Associations and Health Centers. In *Health Policy Seminar Series*. Washington, DC: National Association of Community Health Centers, Inc.

Rosenbaum, S., D. C. Hughes, and K. Johnson. 1988. Maternal and Child Health Services for Medically Indigent Children and Pregnant Women. *Medical Care* 26 (4): 315–32.

Sardell, A. 1988. *The U.S. Experiment in Social Medicine: The Community Health Center Program, 1965–1986*. Pittsburgh, PA: University of Pittsburgh Press.

Schattschneider, E. E. 1960. *The Semisovereign People*. New York: Holt, Rinehart and Winston.

Schorr, L. B. 1988. *Within Our Research: Breaking the Cycle of Disadvantage*. New York: Doubleday.

Starfield, B. 1985. Motherhood and Apple Pie: The Effectiveness of Medical Care for Children. *Milbank Memorial Fund Quarterly* 63 (3): 523–46.

Stevens, R. 1971. *American Medicine and the Public Interest*. New Haven, CT: Yale University Press.

U.S. Congress, Office of Technology Assessment. 1988. *Healthy Children: Investing in the Future*. Washington, DC: U.S. Government Printing Office.

U.S. House of Representatives, Select Committee on Children, Youth, and Families. 1988. *Children and Families: Key Trends in the 1980s*. Staff report. 100th Cong. 2d sess.

Washington Post. 1990. Benefits Grew among Budget Cuts. 3 November, p. A4.

Waxman, H. A. 1989. Kids and Medicaid: Progress but Continuing Problems. *American Journal of Public Health* 79 (9): 1217–18.

Wilson, A. L. 1989. Development of the U.S. Federal Role in Children's Health Care: A Critical Appraisal. In *Children and Health Care: Moral and Social Issues*, ed. L. M. Kopelman and J. C. Moskop. Norwell, MA: Kluwer Academic Publishers.

Health Care and the Homeless:
A Political Parable for Our Time

Bruce C. Vladeck

Abstract. The growth in the number of homeless persons is perhaps the most visible indicator of social disintegration in the 1980s, although health and health care are not the central issues of homelessness. This paper, which draws on the author's experience as chairman of the Committee on Health Care for Homeless People of the Institute of Medicine (IOM), describes what is known about the characteristics of homeless persons and the causes of homelessness, and about the health status of homeless persons, which is often not very good (but not significantly worse, it would appear, than that of other low-income persons). The contemporary history of health services targeted to homeless persons begins with the joint initiative of the Robert Wood Johnson Foundation and the Pew Charitable Trusts in 1985, which became the model for federal support through the Stewart B. McKinney Act of 1987. The McKinney Act, like the IOM report, demonstrates how, in contemporary American politics, there can be widespread political consensus not only about a problem but about solutions, while the resulting policy actions are largely symbolic.

Of all the indicia of social disintegration in the 1980s, none has been more publicly apparent than the extraordinary growth in the number of homeless persons. Partially, no doubt, because of their literal visibility, the homeless appear to have affected public consciousness in a way that other groups of seriously disadvantaged people have not. For once, popular perceptions and underlying realities may be appropriately consonant, since the homeless not only symbolize, but often actually embody, much of what has gone wrong with American society in the last decade. Cutbacks in social programs, changes in the labor market, family disintegration, increased dispersion of income and wealth, and various forms of discrimination are all integrally connected to the plight of the homeless.

It is always troubling, however, to enter into a discussion of homelessness from the perspective of a consideration of health care issues or health care policy. The health problems of homeless persons are formidable and demanding of attention, and the design of intervention strategies invariably raises a host of important and intriguing issues, many of which exemplify broader currents or problems in more general health care policy; but health care is rarely the predominant need of homeless persons, nor are health problems generally their worst problems. Interventions to assist the homeless under the rubric of health care often devote a large share of their resources, necessarily and appropriately, to social services and related issues. Perhaps more importantly, discussions of the health aspects of homelessness run the risk of a detached and clinical focus which loses sight of the more compelling, if more subjective, human aspects of the problem. Information and analysis are appropriate and necessary, but they are no substitute for outrage, and the latter may be a more appropriate response to the realities of the situation.

For fear of outraging the editor of this volume, however, I propose to do the following in this paper: to describe briefly the current phenomenon of homelessness and some of the characteristics of homeless persons; to summarize what is known about the causes of homelessness; and to describe some of the connections between homelessness and health status. That will lead to a brief description of the major private and public health care interventions, followed by some speculation about the politics of homelessness and of health care for the homeless. Much of the material in this paper is drawn from the report of the Committee on Health Care for Homeless Persons of the Institute of Medicine of the National Academy of Sciences (1988), which I chaired, and I will also, in the context of a discussion of the politics of homelessness, make a few observations about the politics of studying the homeless.

The homeless population

No one knows how many homeless people there are in the United States, in part because the homeless are intrinsically difficult to count, in part because estimation of the size of the problem has become a highly politically laden process, and in large part because homelessness is generally not a permanent condition. People become homeless, or cease being homeless, all the time; in the coldest possible terms, we are talking about a flow, not a stock. Thus, the number of persons who are homeless during the course, say, of a year, is far greater than the number of persons who are homeless at any given point in time, and while a significant portion of people who are homeless at any given time have been and will remain homeless for a considerable duration, most of the people who are homeless during a year are homeless for only a few weeks or months at a time.

Nonetheless, we crave numbers, and one plausible estimate suggests that, during 1988, upwards of 700,000 Americans were homeless at any given point in time, as many as two million were homeless during the course of the year, and perhaps as many as six million lived in socioeconomic circumstances that put them at extremely high risk of homelessness (Alliance Housing Council 1988). Certainly, at the bottom of the socioeconomic ladder the boundary between being domiciled and being homeless is extremely thin and highly permeable.

The homeless people one sees on the streets or in transportation terminals, it should be noted, are only a fraction of all the homeless. Indeed, according to the federal statutory definition, the homeless include not only those who lack "a fixed, regular, and adequate nighttime residence," but those whose primary nighttime residence is a shelter, a welfare hotel, other temporary residences, or "a public or private place not designed for, or ordinarily used, as a regular sleeping accommodation for human beings" (Pub. L. No. 100-77). Estimates of the homeless population in any given community are usually derived by counting the shelter population and then estimating the ratio of those in formal shelters to those outside the shelter system; even among the homeless, in other words, there are infinite gradations in the quality of sleeping arrangements, and substantial instability and turnover from one night to the next.

Whatever the actual numbers, there is universal agreement that the number of homeless persons has increased dramatically in the last several years, growing in double-digit proportions from one year to the next. There is also general agreement that the fastest-growing segment of the homeless population is families with young children. Typically, these families consist of a single mother and one or more very young children (although west of the Mississippi two-parent homeless families are reportedly more common—like everything else in contemporary America, a rising tide of social pathology obscures considerable regional and even city-to-city variation).

Nonetheless, it is the single adults, predominantly male, who dominate public consciousness about the homeless. The single homeless tend to be significantly younger than the stereotypical "Skid Row" denizens of older times, with most in their twenties and thirties. They are more likely to be members of racial minority groups than the domiciled population in the communities in which they reside and, perhaps surprisingly, have histories of educational attainment comparable to that of other low-income people of similar ethnicity in their communities. Many have had at least some history of labor force attachment and, contrary to the beliefs of many politicians, a very high proportion have lived for protracted periods in their communities before becoming homeless—with the exception of the Southern California mecca of San Diego, the homeless in most communities are, by and large, longstanding residents of those areas.

These generalizations about longstanding residence and disproportionately minority ethnicity do not apply so readily to one of the fastest-growing and most troubling subgroups in the homeless population, homeless youths and adolescents. Many are runaways; far more may be "throwaways" ejected from family settings. In an ironic commentary on the "successes" of parts of our social welfare system, a growing number have "aged out" of systems for care of the mentally retarded, of juvenile justice systems, or of foster care, and lack the personal skills, economic opportunities, and familial supports to get successfully started in an increasingly Darwinian society. To jump slightly ahead of the outline, the health problems of homeless adolescents are appalling.

The prevalence of identifiable mental illness is far higher among homeless men than it is in the general population, but the consensus of most studies is that that proportion is probably well under half. (For the much smaller population of single homeless women, however, chronic mental illness is overwhelmingly common.) Substance use and abuse are, however, endemic, at least in New York City and some other well-studied communities. The extent to which patterns of drug and alcohol use among homeless individuals predate their homelessness, in contradistinction to developing as part of a shared adaptive pattern of behavior among homeless men, is not known, nor are good comparisons of substance-using behavior between the homeless and domiciled persons of equivalent socioeconomic status even available.

Data on homeless families, whose members are thought to comprise one-third to one-half of all homeless persons, are less extensive, and tend to come from a relatively small number of communities, but there are enough studies to leave room for some controversy. The question, as yet unresolved and possibly unresolvable, is essentially whether those families that become homeless are simply a more or less random sampling of young, extremely low-income mothers with young children, or whether they are more likely than domiciled families to have experienced particular problems, notably multigenerational patterns of intrafamilial violence. In any event, homeless families do tend to be characterized by multigenerational welfare dependency, limited maternal education, and births to very young mothers.

The very rapid increase in the number of homeless persons during the 1980s can be explained by two general metaphors, both of them largely correct. The first, which might be called the ecological model, emphasizes the very rapid increase in the number of poor people in the United States during that decade, the significant shrinkage in the unskilled end of the labor market, and—most centrally—the reduced supply of low-income housing. During the 1980s, the aggregate supply of low-income housing in the United States fell by roughly 2.5 million units at the same time that the demand for such housing, defined in terms of the number of low-income households, was increasing. At this level, the argument is practically syllogistic, though hardly inaccurate: so many people are homeless because there aren't enough homes, and the people without homes lack the financial wherewithal to enter an increasingly expensive housing market.

What might be called the dynamic model takes as a given the facts of the ecological model, but focuses instead on the characteristics of individuals which, in a constrained housing market, precipitate homelessness. Greater emphasis is given to such personal attributes as exacerbations of chronic mental illness, changes in employment status, and family conflict. While this dynamic model diverts attention from the most obvious and most critical public policy interventions that might over time significantly reduce the numbers of homeless persons, it has the advantage of reminding people that homelessness is less a permanent state of being than a dynamic process, in which a large proportion of the individuals or families who are homeless at any given time are likely to experience periods both of being housed and being homeless in the relatively near future.

The dynamic aspect of homelessness is perhaps most crucial in understanding the problems of the chronically mentally ill who, while probably constituting a minority of all homeless persons, occupy so much of the public debate. Policies of deinstitutionalization in state mental health systems have not meant that no one is admitted to mental health facilities any longer. Indeed, while average daily census in some state hospital systems has fallen as much as 90 percent, total admissions have actually increased. What deinstitutionalization really means is shorter stays and rapid discharge, presumably to community-based services and facilities which in principle can provide adequately for most of the chronically mentally ill most of the time.

What renders deinstitutionalization a sham in many parts of the country is simply the absence of such community-based services, with the streets literally serving as the primary alternative. The path of many chronically mentally ill persons, certainly most of those who experience homelessness, is not as neatly unidirectional as the theory would have it, from confined facilities through increasing degrees of freedom in the community. Rather, more typically, it constitutes continual movement through all levels of the system—including the non-system of homelessness. In extreme but hardly rare cases, the metaphor of the revolving door is thus more accurate than that of the progressive continuum.

The interconnectedness of the causes of homelessness with broader social phenomena—and with one another—means that effective policy prescriptions must necessarily deal with broader issues than homelessness per se. Just as it can hardly be coincidental that the greatest acceleration in the size of the homeless population occurred during the apotheosis of the Reagan revolution in domestic social welfare policy, so the changes necessary to substantially reduce the incidence of homelessness will require similarly ambitious social policy innovation—and possibly, as a precondition, similarly dramatic political changes. But the embeddedness of homelessness in broader social forces has strong parallels to, and implications for, the narrower questions of health care and the homeless.

Homelessness and health

Being homeless is bad for your health. All other things being equal, homelessness increases the risk of contracting a range of physical and psychosocial ailments, exacerbates preexisting health problems, and renders more difficult treatment of even relatively treatable conditions.

But all other things are hardly ever equal, and it is difficult to demonstrate, only in part because of data problems, that the health status of homeless persons is substantially worse than that of equally poor, lower-class residents of inner cities or rural areas in which there is considerable homelessness. As a predictor of ill health, poverty remains a far more powerful variable than homelessness per se. That is not to say that the health of the homeless is good, only that the homeless are relatively young and that many low-income people in this society, domiciled as well as homeless, suffer considerable morbidity from conditions that should in principle be treatable.

As a way of organizing the issues it was charged to think about, the Committee on Health Care for Homeless Persons of the IOM developed a three-part paradigm: ill health as a cause of homelessness; homelessness as a cause of ill health; and homelessness as a complicating factor rendering the treatment of illness more difficult (Institute of Medicine 1988: 39–43). None of these categories is empty. Cases of illness or disability-caused unemployment, leading to loss of income and subsequent loss of housing, are numerous and well documented, although their total quantitative impact is hard to estimate. A different instance falling even more squarely into this category is that of the chronically mentally ill individual who decompensates into irrational or violent behavior and is literally ejected from a family domicile.

Homelessness also leads directly to various illnesses of exposure, malnutrition, and, in many shelter settings, infectious diseases, not the least of which is tuberculosis. Each winter, some number of homeless people literally freeze to death. And if the hypothesis suggested above is correct—as I strongly believe to be the case—then the development of certain adaptive behavior patterns, especially among single homeless men, leads to a variety of forms of substance abuse.

Still, it is the third category that, in the aggregate, probably contributes most to excess morbidity and premature mortality among the homeless. To take one dramatic, but hardly uncommon example, the management of insulin-dependent diabetes is effectively impossible when one lacks a safe and secure place to store insulin and syringes, let alone to administer injections. Indeed, it is almost impossible for homeless persons to maintain medication regimens of any kind, including those for psychotropic medications. More generally, think of every physician's—and every grandmother's—prescription for upper respiratory infections: take aspirin or acetaminophen every four hours; drink lots of warm fluids; eat lightly but nutritionally; and get plenty of bed rest. For most homeless persons, none of these is practically possible.

Thus, most providers of health services to the homeless report that most of the illnesses they see are relatively routine, not radically different from what one would encounter in routine general practice in any low-income neighborhood, except, of course, for the higher proportion of psychiatric and substance-related problems. Treatment approaches, however, must often be radically different to accommodate the sorts of difficulties noted above.

The hardest part of health care for homeless people is getting them into treatment in the first place. Homeless persons encounter all the difficulties poor people in general have in getting access to health care, of which the absence of financial means is by far the most important but hardly the only one, but appear to experience additional difficulties in access as well.

Homeless individuals are hardly appealing potential patients to most health care providers, and many, including but not limited to the mentally ill, avoid or resist contact with health professionals or other middle-class strangers. For many individuals, homelessness itself can be interpreted, in a sense, as a result of difficulties in coping with complex and unfriendly bureaucratic systems, and health care often comes in the form of such systems. In general, the experience suggests that, without active outreach efforts, homeless persons will not make extensive use of the health care system.

Similarly, keeping homeless patients in the health care system once they have entered can be a particular challenge for health care providers. In particular, arrangements for follow-up or specialty services, if not provided at the time of initial contact, may pose problems of transportation, scheduling, or other logistical barriers in a population defined by residential instability, and also presume more of a tendency towards compliant behavior than many of the homeless usually exhibit.

Conversely, when homeless people do enter the inpatient health system, it is often difficult to get them out, or at least to get them out in a humane and clinically defensible way. Most discharge planning, of course, rests on the assumption that the patient has a home to return to, and facilities to care for the postacute, convalescent, or chronically ill homeless are scant to nonexistent in most communities. Thus, hospitals that admit homeless patients are often confronted with the choice of letting them remain indefinitely or discharging them literally to the street, and the latter alternative is chosen with disheartening frequency.

Health services to the homeless

Unlike the explosion in the phenomenon of homelessness itself, the development of contemporary services to provide health care to homeless people has a simple and relatively clear genesis. Although there were a few notable precursor programs, the watershed event was the issuance of a request for proposals in late 1983 from the Robert Wood Johnson Foundation and Pew Charitable Trust, to fund programs of health care for the homeless in large cities; eventually, through a competitive process, grants were awarded to 19 of the nation's 50 largest cities. The Johnson-Pew program required that each city's program be governed by a broadly based public/private sector coalition;

that the services supported have a strong outreach component; and that social services, especially those having to do with ensuring homeless people receipt of entitlement benefits for which they were eligible, have a major place in all projects.

Most of the Johnson-Pew projects rely heavily on nurse practitioners and/ or physicians' assistants, as well as nurses and social workers, although all have a considerable physician component, and all emphasize backup arrangements between primary care practitioners in the field and more specialized services at larger health care institutions—backup that often works better on paper than in reality. Most of the work of the Johnson-Pew health care providers involves routine primary care with a particular emphasis on psychiatric and substance abuse counseling, screening for infectious disease and, again, an especially heavy emphasis on social services, especially those having to do with entitlements.

In total, the two foundations contributed $25 million in the period 1985– 1988 to support these programs, in a process that elicited substantial local public and private support as well. To this day, the Johnson-Pew projects remain the backbone of the provision of health care to homeless people in much of the country. In addition to the foundations, they have also been supported by the remarkable institution of Comic Relief, sponsored by professional comedians and their associates, which conducts an annual fundraising special program on cable television and associated local events. Comic Relief has provided important, if secondary, financial support to many of the Johnson-Pew programs; it has also attached to these programs a kind of celebrity, show-business aura of a degree of incongruity somehow prototypical of America in the late twentieth century—*People* magazine meets the bag lady.

The politics of homelessness

As the national foundations so often hope, but as so rarely occurs—at least in the Reagan era—the foundation-sponsored health care for the homeless projects became the model for national policy. In 1987, after several years of nibbling around the edges, Congress enacted the first piece of omnibus legislation directed to the problems of homelessness, the Stewart B. McKinney Homeless Assistance Act (Pub. L. No. 100-77). The health provisions of the McKinney Act were explicitly designed to support the Johnson-Pew programs, along with new programs developed in accordance with the Johnson-Pew model.

Title II of the McKinney Act, which provided for outpatient health services, constituted the first new categorical funding for a health services program in the Reagan era, and that engendered some interesting political byplay. Community health centers funded under Section 330 of the Public Health Service Act had been major victims of Reagan administration cutbacks, and had struggled throughout the decade to maintain some level of services in the face of growing demand from their traditional low-income clientele, constrained Medicaid reimbursement, and reductions in the real level of federal support. Unsurprisingly, in most communities they had done little to reach out to new populations of the homeless, and in the absence of outreach efforts, served relatively few homeless people. They played an extremely limited role in the service coalitions in most of the Johnson-Pew programs, although there were a few notable exceptions, including New York City. But the development of the McKinney Act legislation mobilized the National Association of Community Health Centers, its constituents, and its congressional supporters, especially in the Senate. That, in turn, engendered a counterreaction from many of the Johnson-Pew organizations, which feared being pushed aside as federal funding became available for services they had helped create, often without any substantive help at all from community health centers. The outcome was a compromise, channeling new program funds to the community health centers without giving them as central a role as they had sought, and protecting the roles of most of the Johnson-Pew providers.

More generally, the McKinney Act exemplifies the curious sorts of politics that surround the issue of homelessness in the context of American social welfare policy and politics in the late 1980s. Its scope is broad—encompassing not only outpatient health services but expanded alcohol and drug abuse treatment, transitional housing for displaced families and the chronically mentally ill, community development block grants, expansion of the Section 8 housing voucher program, adult literacy programs, and increased emergency food, shelter, and nutrition programs, along with the inevitable commissions and coordinating councils—but its means are pitifully small, at roughly $500 million a year in authorizations. Strenuously opposed at the outset by the Reagan administration and Republicans at the congressional committee level, it ultimately passed both houses of Congress by wide margins, and was not only signed by the president largely without protest, but then strenuously endorsed a year later by Vice President Bush during his presidential election campaign, perhaps in a preemptive effort to minimize Republican vulnerability on an issue which, in any event, the Dukakis forces were far too inept to exploit.

Homelessness is not, in short, an issue around which there are widespread disagreements about remedies, although on the ideological right there is considerable questioning both of the real significance of the problem and of the appropriateness of any governmental intervention. Nor is there any public argument that it is anything but an objective evil; no one, to my knowledge, has publicly argued that homelessness is good for people, nor even (in the more traditional mode) that the threat of homelessness provides a socially beneficial prod to industriousness among those at the bottom of the labor market—perhaps because among the more visible street homeless population there is so much extremely industrious scavenging, panhandling, and window washing. To be sure, the conservative literature does contain a great deal of victim-blaming: when people are homeless, it's their own fault. But a very broad and reasonably powerful consensus appears to hold that homelessness is bad not only for the individual but for society, that it arises from deep-seated social problems, and that something ought to be done to fix it.

What needs to be done is hardly a great mystery either. More low-income housing must be built; more community-based treatment for mental illness, alcoholism, and drug abuse must be made available; more accessible, effective, and humane social services and emergency services must be provided to those individuals and families most at risk. But in the post-Reagan era, it appears to be sufficient for policymakers to acknowledge all of that, make a few very modest gestures in the right direction, and then move on to something else, confident that there will be no great public outcry against what is essentially a sham being perpetrated. Rhetoric has indeed come to substitute for policy. Perhaps more importantly, the real genius of the 1981 Reagan-Stockman budget and its Gramm-Rudman successor continues to be apparent: Congress can undertake to remedy any evil it wishes, so long as the remedy is budget-neutral.

Thus, two years after the enactment of the McKinney Act the number of homeless people continues to increase, although the issue appears to be of less compelling concern to the public now than it was in the relatively recent past. An increasing proportion of that increasing number of homeless persons now receives formal health services of one sort or another, generally of relatively high quality. We have no evidence as to whether morbidity or mortality is decreasing in that population as a result—on the other hand, there is only so much one can expect from $100 million a year.

The politics of studying homelessness

What the Institute of Medicine ever imagined it could benefit by, or contribute to, a study of the health problems of homeless people is still something of a mystery to me, although throughout its history the IOM has struggled with the tension between its posture of Olympian scientific expertise and its urge to play a larger role among the big boys in the political fray. The actual process by which the IOM became involved was rather straightforward if, in retrospect, somewhat comical. A relatively junior member of the House Committee on Energy and Commerce, excited by the initial publicity surrounding the Johnson-Pew health care for the homeless program in his hometown, where he was already contemplating a run for mayor, managed to attach an obscure amendment to the already obscure Health Professions Training Assistance Act Amendments of 1985, directing the secretary of the Department of Health and Human Services (DHHS) to contract with the IOM for such a study. DHHS did its best to ignore that mandate, hoping it would go away; but IOM staff, eager, at that point in the IOM's history, both for any government contract and for any funding that touched on access issues, kept the issue alive and finessed DHHS into finally letting a contract in late 1986. (That the original congressional sponsor was subsequently indicted on an entirely unrelated matter, thus incurring a fatal blow to his aspirations for higher—or lower—office, is of no immediate relevance to the story.)

Like most IOM "studies," that conducted by the Committee on Health Care for Homeless Persons was not really an investigation in the classic sense of the scientific method at all, but rather a process in which a committee, fed material by its staff, debated the meaning of various research reports and other information. Throughout its life, the committee was hampered, and its work probably distorted, by several staff problems, but push did not really come to shove until well into the final draft of the committee's report. By that point (in the spring of 1988), the obvious policy predilections of a large proportion of the committee's members, combined with the feared political unreliability of the committee's chairman, in the atmosphere of Washington in a presidential election year when the incumbent administration felt justifiably defensive on issues of the homeless, created a degree of nervousness within the IOM and its parent, the National Academy of Sciences. Extensive word-by-word negotiations were conducted between the committee chairman and IOM staff to produce a mutually acceptable set of recommendations.

That compromise was then roundly rejected by a majority of the committee, on the grounds that the negotiated document was both insufficiently specific in its policy recommendations and insufficiently alarmed and passionate in its tone. A further compromise was proposed by the IOM staff: those unhappy with the committee report per se could provide a supplemental statement, which would be published as a nonreviewed statement of opinion in conjunction with the peer-reviewed committee report. The chairman of the outside peer review panel created to review the committee's report enthusiastically endorsed that approach, and such a statement was drafted and agreed to by nine of the thirteen members of the committee, including the chairman.

At that point, the president of the National Academy of Sciences determined that publication of the supplemental statement along with the report was unacceptable, although there was precedent for such an approach, because the supplemental statement was "rhetorical," unscientific, and politically charged. A variety of further compromises were then proposed by the NAS and the IOM, none of them acceptable to the committee. After considerable telephone debate, however, the committee did decide to permit the IOM to proceed with issuance of the report in the form considered acceptable by the NAS—with the addition of a disclaimer on the opening page of the recommendations chapter in which a majority of the committee attacked the recommendations as inadequate—and to pursue publication of the supplemental statement under separate auspices.

The combination of ambivalence and arrogance in the IOM's approach to this issue was perhaps best revealed during the summer of 1988 in a series of telephone calls to the committee's chairman. The IOM was especially eager to conduct a press conference announcing the issuance of the report, but fearful that press coverage would focus (perhaps understandably enough) on the fact that most of the committee's members (a tenth member signed on to the supplemental statement in disgust with the NAS's position) thought the report was inadequate. Thus, the chairman was repeatedly asked if he would be willing to promise not to mention the supplemental statement in a press conference, not to use the "C word" in reference to the NAS's censoring of that statement, and to promise to otherwise behave. The chairman agreed to omit references to the supplemental statement in opening remarks at a press conference, but when he refused to promise not to respond to questions by making reference to the statement, plans for a press conference were finally cancelled. With this background, I must confess that my colleagues on the committee and I took considerable pleasure when the *New York Times* featured the supplemental statement on page 1 in its only coverage of the IOM report (Boffey 1988). The *Washington Post* did not mention the study at all, perhaps from jealousy at the *Times*'s exclusive.

There is a moral to this tale apart from its simple amusement. It has often been observed that Americans are much more comfortable if they can define problems as questions of fact or science rather than as questions of conflicting issues or values, but calling a political issue a question for science doesn't make it one. On the other hand, only scientists really care about the answers to scientific questions. Whether or not the HIV virus causes AIDS is a question best left to the workings of the formal scientific establishment, but how to organize services for AIDS patients—let alone at what level to fund them— is going to get played out in a political process whether or not the scientific establishment expresses an opinion. Nor in this country, as opposed, say, to France, are politicians prone to show much deference to scientists merely because they are scientists when the politicians think the issues belong on their turf.

For an organization like the IOM, this all poses a difficult dilemma, since its charter directs it to the "examination of policy matters pertaining to the health of the public" (Institute of Medicine 1988: ii), but its organization and aspirations lodge it within the National Academy of Sciences and National Research Council, which cling to nineteenth-century distinctions between objective scientific truth and political opinion, and which have long recognized that their political credibility is closely tied to maintenance of that distinction. Once the IOM gets into hard policy questions, it jeopardizes its mantle of scientific authority—not to mention raising questions about the validity of the whole peer-review process which comprises, in fact, the primary objective gesture towards the canons of science. But unless it does, it can't have any fun, nor can its members (many of whom, like myself, aren't scientists by any remote stretch of the imagination) convince their peer groups that they're doing something useful. Better to be unscientific than irrelevant. Or, as I told some of my colleagues during the hullabaloo following release of the supplemental statement, I have no objections to being rolled in a political fight when the other side has more divisions; I just resent being told that it is being done in the name of science. In our secular, technocratic society, that's the equivalent of having your opponent claim that God is on his side.

However good it might make me feel, recounting the silliness surrounding the IOM report on the homeless would be entirely digressive here were it not for the way in which it serves as a kind of microcosm for the politics of homelessness more generally. To paraphrase Dos Passos, ours is increasingly two nations—one educated, affluent, largely white, insured for health care, and domiciled, the other uneducated, poor, disproportionately nonwhite, uninsured, and often homeless—as the result not only of a Darwinian social universe but of conscious public policy choices. That is a fact (whether "scientific" or not) that must be acknowledged if one is serious about doing something to reduce the extent and consequences of homelessness in our society. It is permissible, at least logically, to accept that fact and decide not to do anything about it, or even to conclude that for any of a variety of reasons nothing should be done. But doing so doesn't change the reality. And so long as any of us continue to maintain any illusions about our capacity to influence public policy in an open and still, in many ways, democratic society, the reality of homelessness must stand as recurring evidence of a failure somewhere along the line. The question is not one of facts.

References

Alliance Housing Council. 1988. *Housing and Homelessness*. Washington, DC: National Alliance to End Homelessness.

Boffey, Philip M. 1988. Homeless Plight Angers Scientists. *New York Times*, 20 September, p. 3.

Institute of Medicine, National Academy of Sciences. 1988. *Homelessness, Health, and Human Needs*. Washington, DC: National Academy Press.

Domestic Food Policy in the United States

Michael Lipsky and Marc A. Thibodeau

Abstract. In this paper we review the major outlines of domestic food programs, assess their adequacy, and recommend ways to improve the relationship between food programs and hunger relief. In the Food Stamp Program we treat problems of outreach, coverage and the adequacy of benefits, and rationing access through imposition of costs on recipients. For WIC and commodity distribution programs we also discuss problems associated with the fragmentation of authority and dependence on nonprofit distributors.

Introduction

This paper addresses the delivery of food assistance to individuals and communities in the United States. Our aims are to review the major outlines of food relief programs, assess their adequacy for program recipients, and suggest methods to improve the national response to hunger.

Domestic food assistance policy has been organized historically around three sets of needs. First, the federal government has sought a variety of non-market outlets for surplus agricultural products purchased to maintain farm incomes and prices. Second, it has supplemented the incomes of poor people with food vouchers so that they might have access to an adequate diet. Third, populations considered at nutritional risk have been the focus of special food supplement programs.

Policies responsive to these needs have been subject to several constraints, including the primacy of farm programs if food assistance policy conflicts with them; the tension between program adequacy and cost; and the tension between program outreach and availability on the one hand and program participation by ineligibles on the other.

Programs arising initially out of efforts to support farm incomes or dispose of surpluses purchased to support farm incomes include various institutional feeding programs, of which the School Lunch Program, begun in 1932, is the most notable. The Needy Family Program was the predominant food relief initiative for a decade starting in 1961, and the Temporary Emergency Food Assistance Program revived commodity distribution to households in the 1980s.

The largest income supplement program is the Food Stamp Program, the main avenue for federal food assistance since 1970. The most prominent program to target "at risk" groups for assistance is the Special Supplemental Program for Women, Infants, and Children (WIC). Several other initiatives such as the Child Care Food Program, the Commodity Supplemental Food Program, and other commodity-based programs play a lesser role in meeting specific needs.

We write following an important juncture in food policy development. In 1977, a team of physicians revisited portions of the country that had been found to be rife with hunger and malnutrition a decade earlier (Field Foundation 1977; Citizens' Board 1968). They concluded that hunger had been significantly reduced, due largely to the availability of food stamps. The beginning of the 1980s, however, witnessed the return of widespread domestic hunger, attributable to a deep recession,[1] substantial cuts in food stamps and other social welfare programs,[2] the failure of AFDC payments to keep pace with the rising cost of living,[3] and lagging incomes among the poor that found expression in vast increases in appearances at soup kitchens and government cheese lines.[4]

The period of severe cuts in nutrition programs appears to have abated somewhat, but the structural position of the people who depend on public and private efforts to feed them or to supplement their diets has changed little. Their reliance upon the network of public and private initiatives remains.

------

1. In 1982, the unemployment rate averaged 9.7 percent, representing over 10.7 million people without jobs. Unemployment had increased 2.4 percent over the 1981 rate and 4.1 percent over the 1979 rate. Between 1979 and 1982, the number of unemployed people increased by nearly 4 million (Bureau of the Census 1985: 406).

2. For the years 1982–1985, total cuts in human service programs approached $110 billion. Total outlays for child nutrition programs fell 27.7 percent (Congressional Budget Office 1984: 14; see also Food Research and Action Center 1984a: 27). One million people were dropped from the food stamp rolls, and nearly 20 million people (80 percent of them below the federal poverty level) received less in benefits than before (Legislative Advisory Committee on Public Aid 1984: 6). At the same time, federal support for discretionary (nonentitlement) programs, including commodities, health care, housing, job training, and education, declined sharply. Adjusted for inflation, funding for discretionary programs fell 54 percent between 1981 and 1988, 29 percent if housing is excluded (Center on Budget and Policy Priorities 1988: 5, 7).

3. AFDC benefits declined in real value by more than 35 percent between 1970 and 1988 (Karger and Stoesz 1989: 25). Few states meet the standard of need they have established for residents of their states (Center on Social Welfare Policy and Law 1989: 898).

4. See, for example, Bishop (1983), U.S. Conference of Mayors (1983a, 1983b), and Food Research and Action Center (1984b). Between 1982 and 1986, several dozen reports on hunger (most national in scope) were completed by both public and private sponsors.

Table 1.   Yearly Average Participation in Food Stamps and Commodity Food Distribution (in Millions)

Fiscal Year	Food Stamps	Food Distribution
1961	—	6.38
1963	—	7.01
1964	.36	6.13
1966	1.22	4.78
1968	2.42	3.49
1970	6.46	4.13

Source: McDonald (1977: 4, 12).

Development of food policies

Commodity distribution programs.   Since 1933, the U.S. Department of Agriculture (USDA), armed with the purchasing authority vested in the Commodity Credit Corporation, has bought commodities on the open market for distribution to school and church groups, charitable institutions, local relief agencies, Native American councils, and households.[5] The distribution of surplus commodities was the primary method of delivering food assistance to poor families until 1970 (see Table 1). In recent times, the release of surplus goods to households has been resurrected as an important facet of federal food policy.

Although the ability of surplus disposal efforts to relieve price-depressing farm surpluses found favor with farmers and farm policymakers, its success in alleviating nutritional distress has consistently been disputed by nutritionists and advocates for the poor. It was criticism surrounding the nutritional benefits of the household commodities program that led to its replacement by a food coupon program in 1939 (for a short period) and the Food Stamp Program in the 1970s.

The commodities program was an easy target for nutrition advocates. Initially, the program lacked a stable assortment of foods to hand out and distributed whatever happened to be in surplus. Dietary guidelines did not exist. It was not until 1949 that a relatively stable list of commodities to be purchased was established. Even these commodities, however, were acquired not as mandatory purchases but as price-support purchases. The program was not gov-

---

5. The initial vehicle for distributing foods in this manner was the Agriculture and Food Act of 1935, 7 U.S.C. §612c, 49 Stat. 774. Price support purchases were authorized under the Agriculture Act of 1949, 7 U.S.C. §1431a, 63 Stat. 1057. Distribution authority was expanded under the Older Americans Act of 1965. The distribution of food to congregate feeding sites is regulated by 7 C.F.R. Part 250.

erned by health and nutritional imperatives; rather, it was guided by an agricultural agenda.

During the 1960 presidential campaign, Senator John F. Kennedy observed conditions he found unconscionable among the poor in West Virginia and committed himself to enhancing the federal response to hunger. On the day of his inauguration, his first executive order established the Needy Family Program, which required that a stable supply and expanded list of commodities be made available to households on a monthly basis. That same day he ordered the establishment of pilot food stamp projects.

Criticism of the commodities program did not diminish. The debate focused on the shortage of food availability nationwide, the logistical difficulties of sponsoring the program in rural areas, and the lack of variety and nutritional adequacy of the food packages. Advocates noted that the packages did not include fresh produce, failed to account for religious and cultural preferences, and were excessively bulky. Because participation in the program was a state option, the geographical coverage of the effort was never satisfactory. Even at its peak, the Needy Family Program did not operate in eleven states.

At the same time, bolstered by the apparent success of pilot projects, support for a federal food stamp program grew. Advocates for the poor lauded the payment of vouchers to households as a more nutritionally sound approach. The media, particularly in a landmark documentary produced by CBS in 1968, alerted the public to the pervasiveness of domestic hunger and the inadequacy of federal food policy. Accompanying the criticism of existing policy was the developing view among some agricultural policymakers that increasing consumer purchasing power through food vouchers represented a generally effective, though imprecise, method of reducing surpluses because of the anticipated increase in overall consumption (see, e.g., Paarlberg 1980: 104).

By 1976, fewer than 80,000 people, mostly living on reservations or in trust territories, remained as participants in the direct donation program. By late 1981, however, the farm expansion program of the 1970s (geared to an export market that was diminishing), advances in animal husbandry, and producer-favorable dairy and farm price support programs resulted in billions of pounds of federal food surpluses. Combined with increasing reports of hunger across the country, the surplus held the potential to embarrass a new administration and led President Reagan to reactivate a commodities program for households. Under the aegis of the Special Dairy Distribution Program, local nonprofit institutions received cheese and, later, butter for distribution to needy households.[6]

---

6. Weekly Compilation of Presidential Documents (1981: 1398–99). Other options given consideration by administration and USDA officials involved burying the surplus or dumping it in the ocean. Free distribution was resisted out of fear that it would displace market sales and force the government to purchase more commodities to support prices.

In March 1983, by which time nearly half a billion pounds of dairy products had been distributed, Congress established the Temporary Emergency Food Assistance Program (TEFAP) to formalize the relationship that was being forged among the federal government, the states, and local nonprofit organizations.[7] The program expanded the list of commodities, requiring the distribution of rice, nonfat dry milk, cornmeal, flour, and honey, and made funds available to states and local groups to offset a portion of the costs associated with distribution. In later legislation, Congress required that state-established income eligibility guidelines be used to screen recipients.[8] As of this writing, TEFAP has been reauthorized through federal fiscal year 1990.[9] Since its inception, the staggering total of 6.5 billion pounds of surplus food has been distributed, though recently the pace of distribution has been scaled back due to reductions in surplus stocks.[10]

At its height, TEFAP provided cheese and butter benefitting 19 million people each month, and flour, rice, and cornmeal aiding a much smaller number.[11] This is significantly fewer than the 40 million people deemed eligible for food stamps. It is also important to note that more than half the states established eligibility guidelines well in excess of the food stamp guideline of 130 percent of the poverty level.[12] Thus, only one-third of those eligible for TEFAP receive benefits—an inevitable result, perhaps, of a food program that had its genesis

---

7. Pub. L. No. 98-8, Title II, Temporary Emergency Food Assistance Act of 1983, 98th Cong. 1st sess., 97 Stat. 35–36. See generally Lipsky and Thibodeau (1985, 1988).

8. Pub. L. No. 98-92, Sect. 2, Amendment to the Temporary Emergency Food Act of 1983, 98th Cong. 1st sess., 97 Stat. 608–612.

9. Pub. L. No. 100-435, Hunger Prevention Act of 1988, 100th Cong. 2nd sess., 102 Stat. 1645–1679. For the first time, the secretary of USDA must purchase commodities on the open market, valued at $120 million annually, to ensure an adequate level of distribution for the program. Id. at §214. An additional $40 million must be spent during each of the next three years for foods intended for distribution to soup kitchens and food banks.

10. Over the next two years, it is expected that fewer dairy surplus stocks (but not other food stocks) will be available for distribution than has been the case. During the 1980s, efforts were made to reduce the level of dairy production with the goal of diminishing the government's obligation to purchase surpluses. The Dairy Diversion Program of 1983 lowered dairy price supports and the Dairy Termination Program of 1985 paid farmers to eliminate their dairy herds. Though they were not complete answers to the problem of overproduction (from a market demand perspective), government purchases of dairy surpluses declined from a high of $2.7 billion in 1983 (an elevenfold increase over 1979) to $1.16 billion in 1988. Historically, the dairy sector has proven to be unusually resilient, and it is expected that technological and genetic advances will soon require a high level of government purchases (see CNI Reporter 1989b).

11. For most of the program, approximately 35 million pounds of cheese was released each month in five-pound blocks. The figure of 19 million beneficiaries is calculated by multiplying the 7 million units of cheese distributed by the USDA standard of 2.7 individuals per household. The same method produces the following numbers of beneficiaries for other commodities: nonfat dry milk, 3.4 million; cornmeal, 1.6 million; flour, 1.3 million; rice, 2.7 million.

12. For example, in fiscal year 1985, 25 states maintained an eligibility standard of 150 percent of the poverty level, with nine of those states adopting at 185 percent standard. Since that time, eligibility levels have tended to be more uniform.

in political and market concerns and which lacks the status of a federal entitlement program. The varying eligibility standards maintained by states also
contribute to a problem of distributional equity because the chances of receiving food change drastically depending upon one's residence (see Lipsky
and Thibodeau 1985: 39–47).

Of the four commodity distribution programs to institutions, the School
Lunch Program is the largest (although per meal cost reimbursement represents the bulk of the federal funding commitment), serving approximately
24 million children in 90,500 schools. Half of the children receive free or
reduced-price lunches, fewer than 65 percent of all children who are potentially eligible for them.[13] Reasons that some low-income children do not receive reduced-price lunches include the fact that they live in districts which
have not enrolled in the program or have dropped out due to recent changes
in eligibility (such as the elimination of reduced-price lunches for certain income groups) and administrative impediments (such as the requirement that
a social security number be supplied for all family members).[14]

The School Breakfast Program, intended solely for low-income children,
has far fewer institutional sponsors. Only one-fourth of the needy children
who receive school lunches have access to the breakfast program (Food Research and Action Center 1989a: 5). Even more dramatic is the low participation level of the Summer Food Service Program, a program intended to
provide lunches when school is not in session. In 1983, less than 1.2 million
children participated, more than one-third fewer than participated before the
1981 and 1982 Omnibus Budget Reconciliation acts made it more difficult for
private and nonprofit agencies to sponsor the program. Since those cuts were
made, participation levels in the program have not returned, although the recent authorization of demonstration projects (after a ten-year lapse) for certain
nonprofit institutional providers is promising.[15]

The fact that fewer than 10 percent of the children deemed at risk of nutritional deficiency (according to school lunch program guidelines) participate
in the program might be excused by some on the grounds that the children
are simply not available to school authorities. Various USDA studies, however,
have revealed that school lunch provides poor recipients with at least one-
third of their daily caloric intake. One might be concerned, therefore, about
the dietary gaps many children may experience when they cannot count on
school lunch benefits.

---

13. Prior to the OBRA cuts of 1981, more than 93,000 schools and over 26 million children
were served by the School Lunch Program (Food Research and Action Center 1989a: 2).

14. At this writing H.R. 24, which would eliminate the requirement that social security numbers be supplied for all family members, had passed the House. A measure in the Senate contained
a similar provision.

15. Hunger Prevention Act, supra note 9, §213, 102 Stat. 1658.

The Food Stamp Program.   As noted, the first food stamp program, begun in 1939, was a response to the nutritional inadequacy of the direct donation program. Despite its goal of improving diets, the program was structured as a surplus disposal effort. Recipients received a quantity of coupons for a fee which, theoretically, equalled their normal expenditures for food. Applicants were also given bonus coupons to exchange for foods from a monthly list of surplus commodities made available by the USDA. It was hoped that the absolute level of consumption would be increased as a result. As the perception that it was needed declined, the plan was abandoned in 1943. It was replaced by a restructured commodities program after the war.

As was the case with the earlier program, the 1961 pilot food stamp project included a requirement that the stamps be "purchased," although the price was made equal to only a percentage of normal food expenditures. The purchase requirement was regarded as an incentive to increase consumption and to alleviate the stigma associated with government handouts. The requirement, which some have labeled a self-help provision (Berry 1984), was left intact when the Food Stamp Act of 1964 was passed. The twin congressional goals of the three-year program were the reduction of the nation's food surpluses and the promotion of nutritional well-being (McDonald 1977: 7). Federal controls were minimal, and counties retained the option to choose either a commodities program or a food stamp program. Individual states set the cutoff level for food stamp eligibility.

Concern for hunger in the late 1960s, however, generated momentum for increased federal intervention.[16] In 1969, President Nixon declared that food stamps were to have priority over direct commodity distribution, that certain categories of poor people should receive free stamps, and that benefit levels should be raised significantly. These changes were approved in the 1971 amendments to the act, an act which also set federal eligibility standards. Benefit levels doubled under the legislation, and participation soared (McDonald 1977: 14; Berry 1984: 68–74, 82). Nevertheless, the choice of food assistance program was left a matter of local option. It was not until 1974 that the Food Stamp Program became a mandatory, nationwide effort. The final major change to the program came in 1977 with the elimination of the purchase requirement for all recipients. Since that time, benefit levels have been increased and then lowered, participation has expanded and then contracted, and eligibility standards have been liberalized and then tightened. The essential features of the program—mandatory state participation, nationally uniform benefit levels, and stamps at no dollar cost to recipients—have remained intact.

---

16. Among events that motivated these calls were the CBS documentary on domestic, rural hunger, the Citizen's Board Report referenced earlier, and the Poor Peoples' March on Washington.

Benefit levels are currently based on the Thrifty Food Plan (TFP), developed by the USDA in 1965 and adjusted only slightly since then. The TFP reflects a calculation of the cost of maintaining a family of four on an emergency, temporary basis at minimum nutrient levels. The plan assumes that 30 percent of a household's income (in addition to food stamps) will be spent on food, an indirect "purchase" requirement. Although the TFP represents the official cost of bare maintenance, Congress accepted the president's recommendation in 1981 to reduce food stamp allotments to 99 percent of the value of the plan. Allotments were restored to 100 percent in 1984, and, to the surprise of many, recent legislative changes have mandated an increase to 103 percent by 1991.[17]

Much discussion has concerned the extent to which the TFP is adequate beyond an emergency basis, and its premise that 30 percent of household income would be spent on food in light of the 35–40 percent loss of purchasing power experienced by AFDC recipients since 1970.[18] Criticism has also centered on the appropriateness of its sociological and behavioral assumptions: standardized household needs and standardized food price access nationwide, fully rational food purchase and consumption practices, and a bare minimum of waste in food preparation. The TFP further assumes a standard mother/father/two-children family with no pregnancy or developing child, a family member with time to prepare all meals from scratch, and adequate transportation to take advantage of low price opportunities.

Various studies have demonstrated that families must spend well in excess of the amounts available through food stamps in order to achieve the nutrient value they should receive under the TFP.[19] Typically, the excess expenditure equals 30 percent—ironically, an amount equivalent to the 30 percent income assumption incorporated in the TFP.

One apparent advantage of the Food Stamp Program for low-income recipients has been that its benefits are indexed to inflation, although this feature is somewhat compromised because adjustments to benefits usually lag behind price increases by fifteen months. Combined with the decline of AFDC benefits and other income, the ability of food stamp recipients to purchase adequate amounts of food has become increasingly problematic, all the more so

---

17. Hunger Prevention Act of 1988, supra note 9, §120, 120 Stat. 1655. On average, the value of stamps received by households will increase by $9 per month.

18. In 1988, the average AFDC benefit level was only 47 percent of the official poverty level. In 39 states, the combined AFDC and food stamp grant was less than 75 percent of the federal poverty level (Center on Social Welfare Policy and Law, 1989: 896).

19. For example, the government's last major nutrition study, the 1977 National Food Consumption Survey, indicated that few households achieve dietary sufficiency under the TFP. "USDA found [in the consumption survey] that 88% of individuals purchasing food valued at the equivalent of the Thrifty Food Plan were eating diets that did not meet the Recommended Dietary Allowances set by the government" (Physician Task Force on Hunger 1986: 38).

when one considers that in constant terms, the value of annual benefits received per participant fell from $629 to $602 between 1981 and 1985 (Center on Budget and Policy Priorities 1987). Those cuts have never been restored, and the real purchasing value of stamps has not increased noticeably since 1985. National studies of hunger have consistently pointed out that many households run out of stamps 5–10 days before the end of the benefit month.

The rate of participation has been a source of concern throughout the life of the program. Currently, approximately 19 million people receive benefits, representing about 50 percent of all eligible recipients. Significantly lower percentages are recorded for the elderly (less than 40 percent) and single-member households (30–35 percent). In 1980, the program reached 68 out of every 100 people at or below the poverty line (the cutoff for eligibility is 130 percent of the poverty line). By the end of 1985, only 59 out of every 100 people were reached (Food Research and Action Center 1988).[20]

The size of the participating population is closely connected to eligibility standards. The 1981 OBRA cuts eliminated approximately one million non-elderly food stamp recipients by basing eligibility on gross income rather than on a calculation that allowed consideration of work-related expenses, excess shelter costs, and other deductions. This caused a reduction of benefits to millions of other recipients as well. These changes have been uniformly identified as prime contributors to the increase in hunger nationwide during the 1980s.

To increase participation, Congress historically has funded outreach efforts under the Community Food and Nutrition Program (CFNP). These efforts ended in 1981 when the federal government removed the condition that states sponsor affirmative outreach as part of their administration of the program and stopped funding outreach programs. Outreach efforts are particularly important because lack of information regarding the program and doubts as to eligibility have been identified as the most common reasons why households do not participate in the program.[21] In 1986, some funding for CFNP was restored, though the level of funding ($1.5 million) permits only the sketchiest of state outreach efforts. Few states supplement outreach funds in a meaningful way. Some federal money has been made available to sponsor demonstration outreach projects by nonprofit organizations, though it is not expected that these projects will be operating in more than a dozen states.

---

20. See Physician Task Force (1986: 44) for a breakdown and discussion of the decline in participation per year. See also Center on Budget and Policy Priorities (1986). Low participation is a particular affliction of the rural poor, a group which records only 44 percent participation (Public Voice for Food and Health 1989).

21. See, e.g., Coe (1983). USDA-sponsored studies have reached the same conclusion and have also found that informational barriers are more profound among the elderly (see General Accounting Office 1986).

Targeted nutrition programs.   Low-income pregnant and postpartum mothers and their children are the beneficiaries of the Special Supplemental Program for Women, Infants, and Children (WIC).[22] Begun in 1972 as a pilot project, the program delivers benefits nationwide through more than 1,600 local government agencies and as many as 7,500 special WIC outlets such as social service agencies and neighborhood health clinics. Eligibility qualifications are based on a combination of medical and income guidelines. Because WIC is not an entitlement program, however, eligibility does not guarantee that a qualified mother will be enrolled.

Benefits are delivered to recipients in three ways: food packages containing items with a prescribed nutrient content distributed by WIC outlets; vouchers for infant formula, cheese, iron-fortified cereal, and fruit juices for redemption in retail stores; and direct dairy distribution to the homes of recipients. Apart from the targeted population, WIC is distinguished from other foods programs by health care and nutrition education components. Women are referred to a WIC agency only if they are determined to be at nutritional risk by a qualified health professional. Follow-up medical evaluations are provided periodically. Preventive nutrition education is mandatory, with one-sixth of all program funds allocated for this purpose.

Over its eighteen-year history, the WIC budget has increased from $20 million to more than $2 billion. Current budgetary levels, however, permit only 45–50 percent of eligible mothers and but 35 percent of eligible children to be reached (Center on Budget and Policy Priorities 1989; Food Research and Action Center 1989b). Despite strong national and local organizing efforts, only a dozen states supplement their federal grants in order to expand the number of eligibles served.

Many policy analysts believe that it is particularly shortsighted to deny WIC funding to cover the entire eligible population. WIC not only impacts on the fetal death rate, but it also affects the incidence of low birthweight and premature birth. The cost of WIC is more than recovered by the reduction in postnatal hospital costs. Evidence suggests that every dollar spent on WIC results in a $1–$3 savings in Medicaid outlays.[23]

The Commodity Supplemental Food Program (CSFP), targeted to aid postpartum mothers and the elderly, is structured on medical and income guidelines similar to those for WIC. A monthly package of surplus commodities based on a carefully drawn dietary plan is distributed to recipients by a private,

---

22. WIC was an amendment to the Child Nutrition Act of 1966. See P.L. 92-433, §9, 86 Stat. 729.

23. See Food Research and Action Center (1989b) for a report summarizing research findings on WIC. USDA has sponsored studies of the program and has reported marked decreases in hospitalizations due to low birthweights, premature births, and other conditions related to inadequate prenatal care.

nonprofit sponsor agency. Although CSFP has a positive impact on the major health indicators for the groups it serves, the program has never been authorized beyond a few nonprofit outlets nationwide.

Ongoing issues

Food policy is delivered to communities in two ways: through quasi-income transfers (the Food Stamp Program), and through public and nonprofit agencies, mostly in the form of surplus commodities. Each of these approaches has its characteristic issues.

The Food Stamp Program delivers aid in the form of cash substitutes. Thus the problems of policy delivery tend to be those associated with cash entitlement programs: outreach, coverage, and adequacy of benefits; limiting program access through the imposition of costs on recipients; and managing the problem of ineligibles on the rolls.

Virtually every other food policy is delivered through a series of public and nonprofit organizations whose acceptance of federal feeding initiatives and whose capabilities in running programs to feed those deemed needy critically affect individual access to benefits. Many of these programs also depend on vigorous state action to achieve results. These facets of food policy delivery mean that many benefits are uncertainly available to people in need because they are dependent on the infrastructure available in different states and localities.

Food stamps.   A major disincentive to food stamp participation disappeared when the purchase requirement was eliminated during the Carter administration. Significant underenrollment, however, continues to exist for many demographic groups. No single barrier accounts for these low participation rates, although there is agreement that among the barriers are the administrative difficulties of enrollment and of maintaining registration, ignorance regarding eligibility, and the low benefit levels received in comparison to the detailed inquiry and paperwork burdens one experiences when applying for stamps. Continuing stigma associated with food stamp usage also plays a role.[24]

Problems of negotiating bureaucratic hurdles and paying high "prices" in the form of administrative hassles are getting worse. In this decade, USDA and congressional initiatives have been designed to force states to pay closer attention to administrative practices that may result in errors of leniency toward food stamp recipients (Brodkin and Lipsky 1983). They have done this by imposing severe sanctions for excessively high error rates and by offering sub-

---

24. A review of the literature on low participation in the Food Stamp Program is found in Physician Task Force (1986: 54–83).

stantial incentives to states that meet the target rates.[25] These initiatives typically result in states adopting practices that increase the difficulties of getting on the rolls. It is revealing that only for the coming year (FY 1990) will USDA finally begin to hold states accountable for errors of *underissuance* to recipients.[26]

High food stamp error rates are not helped by continual food stamp revisions (nearly 200 separate regulatory changes have been introduced this decade), which require states to perpetually retrain food stamp workers and revise eligibility systems.[27] Between 1982 and 1988 (the period for which final error rates have been announced), few states have been able to meet or improve on the target rate in any given year.[28]

An important yet subtle concern is the development of administrative practices and legislative demands on administration that result in "bureaucratic disentitlement." The term refers to administrative changes that reduce the number of participants by making participation more difficult—as did monthly budget reporting, and as do mandatory work requirements. The term applies as well to reductions in the number of participants as states, faced with increasing financial sanctions and lowered tolerances for food stamp error rates, become more zealous in guarding the gates to admission. Verification extremism is the result. Disentitlement should be of particular concern because it takes place in the half-light of administrative details and procedures,

---

25. In 1981, the Food and Nutrition Service imposed $25 million in sanctions on fourteen states for overpayments. For 1985, 45 states and three jurisdictions were assessed penalties of over $210 million (Food Research and Action Center 1987: 1). Due to the extraordinary sanction levels, Congress authorized studies of the quality control (QC) system by USDA and the National Academy of Sciences (NAS).

The reports were released in May 1987 and came to different conclusions over the efficacy of QC policy. The USDA urged no changes to the current system, as the agency believed it promoted efficiency and served as a valuable management tool. The NAS, on the other hand, found that program administration was not enhanced and that the method of assessing penalties was biased heavily against states (see Office of Analysis and Evaluation 1987; Panel on Quality Control of Family Assistance Programs 1987).

The title of the NAS report was prophetic, as Congress adopted many of the NAS's recommendations and rolled back sanction amounts that had been imposed for 1986 and 1987 (see General Accounting Office 1987). In 1988, nine states will be sanctioned with potential liabilities of $36 million. Significantly, however, Congress failed to accept the NAS recommendation to alter the definition of sanctionable overpayments to exclude from the error rate cases which, based on information available to the state at the time, were eligible for benefits but later were found to be ineligible. Such a policy fosters verification extremism among states, significantly increasing the verification burdens imposed on recipients (see Center for Social Welfare Policy and the Law 1989: 901).

26. Hunger Prevention Act, supra note 12, §320, 102 Stat. 1661.

27. Regulatory changes have been a hallmark of the program during the 1980s. During one 30-month period at the beginning of the decade, the Food and Nutrition Service initiated 90 major regulatory changes (see Physician Task Force 1986: 109).

28. In this period, no industrialized state was able to meet the target error rates for any year. Only the Dakotas and Nevada have been able to earn incentive payments for their low rates.

and is debated over issues of efficiency, program accuracy, and management rather than of benefits, needs, and deprivations.

USDA has imposed a number of administrative requirements which have had the effect of "churning" many individuals off the rolls for short periods for any of a number of petty offenses (Lipsky 1984). The violations by recipients are normally small, and in an administrative environment more oriented toward getting food to the hungry, they would not result in the interruption of benefits. Inappropriate terminations for technical reasons impair the delivery of benefits and threaten many recipients whose needs have not changed. Nor are increasing barriers to participation in food programs confined to food stamps. School lunch administration has been plagued by official federal concerns over the possible cheating of parents in applying for school lunches, and the imposition of administrative barriers to participation that take the form of greater scrutiny of eligibility.

No doubt systems to deter cheating and maintain administrative integrity are necessary and appropriate in all public programs. But not every program should have the same degree of administrative effort dedicated to fiscal integrity and quality control because programs differ in the stakes involved and in the likelihood of transgressions, and because the tighter the controls, the greater the deterrence to participation. These questions of proportion arise in considering the heavy requirements associated with enrolling for food stamps, the actual monetary value at risk for states in issuing stamps inappropriately, and the likelihood that certain members of society will cheat.

Potential elderly recipients, for example, report that the high cost to them in terms of travel, waiting time, bureaucratic hassles, and periodically going to the welfare office to fill out a complete reregistration form when their status has not changed (they live on fixed incomes) deters them from participating in food stamps when the value of the stamps is fairly low. These are people who are at high risk of undernutrition. Simplified registration and reregistration procedures would be highly salutary for this population, and would provide savings in state administrative costs with little likelihood of rampant cheating.

A provision introduced by the Food Security Act of 1985, which requires food stamp recipients to participate in employment and training programs, is another policy designed to impose additional costs on recipients seeking hunger relief.[29] This initiative draws on the appeal of the self-help work ethic

29. Many states are invoking noncompliance with employment and training requirements to eliminate recipients from the food stamp rolls for a period of up to two months. For example, for the first two quarters of fiscal year 1989, three times as many people in Maryland were sent sanction notices when compared to recipients required to participate in the program who actually did participate. Nationally, under 500,000 people who were required to participate did so, while more than 160,000 were sent sanction notices, a rate of approximately 33 percent, with ten states exceeding 50 percent.

and public support for work initiatives in AFDC to justify the imposition of barriers to an entitlement program. To draw from the AFDC experience, however, only work requirements accompanied by significant allocation of resources to assist recipients with training, education, and child care stand a chance of assisting unemployed people to get off the rolls and remain in good jobs. States have complained that federal food stamp employment and training resources are grossly inadequate.[30] Nevertheless, thousands of recipients have been forced from the rolls for failure to fulfill mandatory participation requirements.

One recalls that the purchase requirement was eliminated more than a decade ago because it hindered participation and thus detracted from a primary purpose of the Food Stamp Program. Work requirements in food stamps have the same effect unless they are designed (as they currently are not) to raise recipients' income so that the marginal benefits of working are sufficiently higher than the increased costs of participation.[31] Most significantly, mandatory work and other requirements imposed on recipients of food stamps and other welfare benefits shift the fundamental premise of welfare programming from one based on financial and categorical entitlement to one based on the fulfillment of contract terms with the state. It is revealing that the "level of effort" required of recipients in some employment and training programs is tied to the value of the food stamps they receive.

Other food programs.   Problems associated with food policy delivery outside of food stamps may first be suggested by the sheer number of government agencies and private organizations charged with responsibility for service delivery. State agencies administer a dozen food and nutrition programs through more than 160,000 school districts, hospitals, day care centers, summer camps, WIC offices, and emergency feeding organizations. This is an extraordinary number of organizations with which to charge the responsibility for feeding the hungry in the United States.

There is no single agency or place in the federal, state, or local political structure that assumes jurisdiction over food relief efforts. Ten congressional

---

30. In partial response to these criticisms, Congress has made available $160 per month per dependent in child care expenses, effective 1 July 1989. See Hunger Prevention Act, supra note 9, §404(c), 102 Stat. 1666.

31. Although states have been required to operate food stamp and employment training programs since April 1986, state performance is not judged on the success of the program in placing recipients in jobs; indeed, there is no place on USDA reporting forms for states to indicate whether they have had any success in job placement. Though performance standards based on "employment outcomes" were scheduled to go into effect in January 1991, the administration's recent budget proposal recommended that standards be delayed until October 1993. One may then question whether such employment programs are more symptomatic of a shift in the political mood in favor of "make work" programs than a reasoned attempt at welfare reform, as supporters have argued.

committees, five separate federal departments, and one independent federal agency (FEMA) lay claim to a slice of the food program pie. As a result, the often conflicting interests of agribusiness, farmers, health care and welfare policymakers, and food relief efforts abroad compete for influence and advantage.

Despite the array of programs that have arisen, city by city, supported by a combination of federal, state, and private funds, there is little public infrastructure charged with managing the issue of hunger. Public officials are reluctant to institutionalize emergency relief programs because they fear people who use such services will become more dependent than ever. In short, there is only an uneven, uncoordinated structure that takes responsibility for providing relief when people declare themselves, for whatever reason, to be hungry.

Another critical concern in supplementary food policy delivery is the unequal distribution of supplementary feeding agencies. Whether one receives this type of assistance depends on whether one resides in a place which has a program. Does your school system have a school lunch and breakfast program? Does your county have a WIC program? Does your state supplement its WIC grant? Has the state in which you live been able to locate a community organization in your area able and willing to distribute cheese and butter? Answers to these questions determine access to supplementary food relief. Throughout the nation, people equally needy by virtue of low income or hunger have radically different access to assistance based on local governmental and private capacity to field feeding policies.

An immediate objection to this critique is that access to social welfare benefits in the American federal system generally involves inequalities because such policies are properly determined by the plans and initiatives of the states. Two responses are in order. First, other social welfare programs have been recognized as national in consequence and effect, yet have not been subject to the unevenness of state responsibility and initiative. Food stamps and social security are but two programs with federal standards and scales. Moreover, even in AFDC, the model of a program based on a state's right to set standards has been moving in the direction of greater uniformity of scope and coverage over the years.

Second, there is a critical distinction between national policy to let states determine their own standards for implementing national social welfare policies and dependence of the population of states on the existence, enthusiasm, and capacity of private nonprofit organizations and local public agencies to provide feeding services. One can respect the federal compact with the states which has led to some variability in state AFDC plans and still reject the idea that people should go hungry in some parts of the country because food banks do not exist in their areas, or because school boards cannot or will not provide school lunches or breakfasts to eligible children. The availability and level of commitment of the voluntary sector is not a matter of public policy in the various states, but at best is a matter of divergent political, cultural, and social developments that have little basis in public policy or prior legislation.

Other important barriers to equitable treatment of people similarly situated may be identified in food policy delivery. Mothers and infants eligible for WIC are regularly denied enrollment in the program because funds are limited and full funding for all eligible citizens, including those in categories most at risk of nutritional deficits, has never been made available by Congress. Peculiarly, *when* you happen to be in need may also determine whether you receive services, because many WIC programs regularly close off intake when they project that current clients will utilize available annual funds.

TEFAP has proven to be another program for which the timing of one's need may affect receiving assistance. More than twenty states substantially reduced their surplus food distribution in the summer of 1985, for example, as they projected they had used up funds made available to reimburse them and local feeding organizations for expenses associated with TEFAP distribution. In addition, the frequency of state distributions and the geographical reach of the program within states is such that access to commodities has become a game of chance.

A word should be said for the public role in supporting feeding efforts by the private, nonprofit sector. The rise of food banks over the last decade in response to the unmet needs of the hungry in local communities has been critical in filling some of the gaps in public food relief efforts. The Second Harvest network of 200 food banks and affiliates which serve nearly 40,000 charitable feeding organizations nationwide, the Self-Help and Resource Exchange (SHARE) program, and other unaffiliated efforts have been impressively successful in soliciting contributions from food processors, wholesalers, farmers, and supermarkets and in engaging in selective bulk food buying (Crawford 1989). Run with small paid staffs and the energies of thousands of volunteers working for the satisfaction of helping their neighbors or the promise of a bag of groceries, these organizations help supply the soup kitchens, brown bag programs, and other feeding activities at the local level.

Although the role of these programs has been a worthy one and their potential remains high, they are ultimately limited by the depth of the hunger problem, their dependence on volunteers, and the availability of government and food industry surpluses. Special tax advantages to corporations have encouraged donations of retail products, and TEFAP has made important contributions to private feeding initiatives by providing reliable sources of protein to programs otherwise dependent on the grab bag of food industry excesses and waste. Nevertheless, a mistaken premise in policy planning holds that the nonprofit sector is in a position to assume responsibility for the large number of people unserved or underserved by federal food programs.

Directions for the future

The United States has the means to develop appropriate programs to improve the food intake of the poor. Realization of the full potential of these programs would go far to alleviate hunger. Yet food and nutrition advocates are under no illusions concerning public support for food and nutrition policy. "Safety net" feeding programs were cut in the early 1980s by Congress and the president, and they may well be cut again as the budget deficit dominates federal decisionmaking. Nevertheless, advocates have been able to develop and nurture a core of bipartisan congressional support for hunger-related issues.

A great deal of progress in food and nutrition could be achieved through the expansion and refinement of existing programs. Food stamp benefits should be increased to match the cost of providing for a full month of food purchases minimally required to provide adequate nutrition. Asset limits (which often make the recently unemployed ineligible for benefits) should be raised to increase the pool of eligible recipients. State AFDC and other welfare programs should be indexed to inflation. Federal policy has recognized the special vulnerability of pregnant women and infant children. Yet the WIC program remains poorly funded relative to declared need and should be made an entitlement program. Consideration should be given as well to providing pregnant women with an enhanced food stamp benefit during the term of pregnancy. The incidence of pregnancy positively influences the level of benefits in all welfare programs, with the exception of food stamps. Allowing for benefits for pregnant women in this manner would be simple to implement, of moderate cost, and would well serve a primary purpose of the program.

A significant aspect of domestic food policy has been the provision of commodity benefits. These valuable supplemental programs depend on a vast array of public feeding agencies and nonprofit organizations willing to make foods available. Because supplemental feeding programs are now unevenly available, an improved feeding policy requires the nationalization of WIC, financial incentives for localities to increase participation in school breakfast and other child nutrition initiatives, increased funding for TEFAP to permit more even distribution of commodities to households, and continued emergency funding to respond to needs that remain unmet by the patchwork of other feeding initiatives. It also follows that the federal government should promote the orderly growth of food banks and other private emergency feeding organizations by providing technical assistance and seed money to help fill in the network of organizations available to meet supplementary food needs.

In the past, the federal government, through the Community Food and Nutrition Program of the Office of Economic Opportunity, and later through the Community Services Administration, played an honorable role in advancing awareness of hunger issues and in facilitating local initiatives. These initiatives were both eliminated in the OBRA of 1981. They returned five years later in a reduced form, but are threatened once again. The fiscal year 1990 Department of Health and Human Services budget proposal would eliminate the Community Services Block Grant. Outreach efforts to maintain and expand participation are particularly warranted in the Food Stamp Program because it is an entitlement program. The low participation rate in food stamps relative to the pool of eligibles blurs the distinction between the concepts of entitlement rights and discretionary rights in welfare programming and dilutes the value and purpose of the entitlement benefit.

Community food advocacy continues, of course, as private sources have partly filled the gap, and the heightened public awareness of hunger has directed the attention of community agencies and activists to this problem. People who provide direct services, however, have difficulty playing advocacy roles. Ideologically, they are often torn because they provide necessary, temporary, emergency assistance and fear that their efforts represent short-term solutions that allow society to avoid confronting more comprehensive policy initiatives. They often have to spend most of their time running their organizations and maintaining systems of assistance when it is clear that energies need to be devoted to political activity at city, state, and national levels. Strident political activity, however, may serve to alienate corporate support, a matter of particular concern to the food bank network, which depends on national companies to supply about 40 percent of all food distributed. Nonprofit providers of food relief are concerned that their criticisms of state and local officials may hurt them when contracts are renegotiated. Fractionalization among nonprofit providers inhibits the development of a stable advocacy strategy.[32]

Advocates also confront the structural problem of acting in local arenas, and thus are a fragmented force when they try to gather their concerns and influence at the national level. For more than a decade, nutrition advocates have sought unsuccessfully to persuade Congress to enact an annual national nutrition survey to provide an ongoing capacity to record progress and identify continuing sources of need.[33] Such a survey would provide visibility to the issue of nutritional adequacy and a rallying point for food advocates, much as the "poverty line" (however inadequately drawn) allows advocates and

---

32. In some metropolitan areas, political considerations have informed decisions of access to and control over food relief. Control of surplus food distribution and antihunger programs represent sources of patronage and influence over critical resources in low-income communities. See, e.g., Thibodeau (1985).

33. Although important monitoring activities do take place, in particular the National Health and Nutrition Examination Survey (HANES) and the Nationwide Food Consumption Survey (NFCS), no survey identifies the populations at risk of undernutrition or points to policy options based on statistical experience (see Hirschoff 1988: 5).

planners to chart success or failure by legitimate measure. The initiative is important for providing not only ongoing monitoring but also the basis for a continuing politics of nutrition advocacy.

It appeared that the efforts of advocates had borne fruit at the end of 1988 with congressional passage of the National Nutritional Monitoring and Related Research Act of 1988. The act called for the implementation of a joint DHHS and USDA monitoring and research program to extend over a ten-year period. Technical assistance was to be provided to states to aid local monitoring efforts. The act emphasized the need to study groups at high risk of undernutrition and certain geographical areas and was expected to cost $250,000 annually. At the outset of his administration, President Reagan indicated that evidence of domestic hunger was purely anecdotal and scoffed at the charge that federal programs were not adequate to meet domestic needs. In his final days in office, the president declined the opportunity to expand the body of knowledge regarding domestic nutrition problems and pocket-vetoed the legislation.

It is time that concerted efforts be made to place food programs on a sounder, nutrition-based footing. Although hunger is a health problem and a poverty problem, no presumption is made in government food policy that assistance programs should be designed with public health goals in mind. Food stamp benefit levels, for example, are informed by assumptions about the purchasing power needed to acquire a minimally adequate diet. Commodity programs are highly responsive to market forces. Even though WIC is intended to respond to an urgent medical need, the lack of an entitlement to benefits reflects an incomplete commitment to child and maternal health.

It is also time to withdraw USDA's authority (through its Food and Nutrition Service) to administer the nation's child nutrition programs—the Food Stamp Program and WIC. That USDA has been delegated authority to run these programs is reflective of a period when the science of nutrition was in its infancy and nutritional and health goals were greatly subordinate to the perceived needs of the national farm economy. Historically, USDA has been highly responsive to the complaints of farmer, producer, and processor interests, with little appreciation for the needy when the interests of the two conflict. The struggle between agricultural economists and nutritionists within USDA has lasted for more than fifty years. Bureaucratic victories for nutritionists have been few.[34]

It is instructive that few states administer nutrition programs through departments of agriculture; rather, school nutrition programs are run through departments of education, WIC through departments of public health, and

---

34. See, e.g., CNI Reporter (1989a: 4–5) for a summary of conflict. It was in 1939 that USDA released its first publication concerning the role of nutrition in health.

food stamps through departments of welfare. The federal government would be wise to follow the state pattern. USDA has unrivaled expertise in managing commodity purchase, storage, and distribution activities. The agency's role should be limited to providing those support services.

These efforts should be part of a broader national goal to ensure the adequacy of diets. The current commitment to this goal is sorely lacking. As a result, the continued vigor of nutrition policy will fall on the small group of people and organizations that make adequate food policy their central concern, and their ability to expand public awareness of the ongoing hunger crisis for millions of Americans.

References

Berry, Jeffrey M. 1984. *Feeding Hungry People: Rule-Making in the Food Stamp Program*. New Brunswick, NJ: Rutgers University Press.

Bishop, Kathryn. 1983. *Soup Lines and Food Baskets: A Survey of Increased Participation in Emergency Food Programs*. Washington, DC: Center on Budget and Policy Priorities.

Brodkin, Evelyn, and Michael Lipsky. 1983. Quality Control in AFDC as an Administrative Strategy. *Social Service Review* 57: 1–34.

Bureau of the Census, U.S. Department of Commerce. 1985. *Statistical Abstract of the United States*. Washington, DC: U.S. Government Printing Office.

Center on Budget and Policy Priorities. 1986. An Analysis of Changes in Food Stamp Participation. Washington, DC: Center on Budget and Policy Priorities.

———. 1987. Fact Sheet: Analysis of the President's June 11, 1987 Statement. Washington, DC: Center on Budget and Policy Priorities.

———. 1988. The New Reductions in Low-Income Programs in FY 1988. Washington, DC: Center on Budget and Policy Priorities.

———. 1989. *Holes in the Safety Net*. Washington, DC: Center on Budget and Policy Priorities.

Center on Social Welfare Policy and Law. 1989. Welfare Law in 1988. *Clearinghouse Review* 9 (January).

Citizens' Board of Inquiry into Hunger and Malnutrition in the United States. 1968. *Hunger USA*. Boston: Beacon Press.

CNI Reporter. 1989a. Nutrition Waits 50 Years in Wings of Food Policy. 25 May, pp. 4–5.

———. 1989b. Dairy Termination Program Produced Mixed Results. 20 July, pp. 4–5.

Coe, Richard. 1983. Nonparticipation in Welfare Programs by Eligible Households: The Case of the Food Stamp Program. *Journal of Economic Issues*, December.

Congressional Budget Office. 1984. *The Combined Effects of Major Changes in Federal Taxes and Spending Programs Since 1981*. Washington, DC: Congressional Budget Office.

Crawford, Lynda. 1989. Food Banking: Who Benefits? *Seeds* 11: 12–18.

Field Foundation. 1977. Physician's Report on Field Investigations. New York: Field Foundation.

Food Research and Action Center. 1984a. *Hunger in the Eighties: A Primer*. Washington, DC: Food Research and Action Center.

———. 1984b. Still Hungry: A Survey of People in Need of Emergency Food. Washington, DC: Food Research and Action Center.

———. 1987. *Foodlines*. Washington, DC: Food Research and Action Center.

———. 1988. Options for Expanding and Improving Federal Nutrition Programs. Washington, DC: Food Research and Action Center.

———. 1989a. Fact Sheets on Federal Food Programs. Washington, DC: Food Research and Action Center, March.

———. 1989b. WIC Misses Half of Eligible Population. *Foodlines* 7 (August).

General Accounting Office. 1986. Overview and Perspectives on the Food Stamp Program. Washington, DC: GAO.

———. 1987. *National Academy of Sciences' Recommendations on the Sanctions Backlog*. Washington, DC: GAO.

Hirschoff, Paula M. 1988. Hunger: Federal Policy Today. *Hunger Notes*, September.

Karger, Howard J., and David Stoesz. 1989. Welfare Reform: Maximum Feasible Exaggeration. *Tikkun*, March/April.

Legislative Advisory Committee on Public Aid, State of Illinois. 1984. *The Impact of Federal Budget Cuts in Illinois*. Springfield: Illinois Department of Public Aid.

Lipsky, Michael. 1984. Bureaucratic Entitlement in Social Welfare Programs. *Social Service Review* 58: 3–27.

Lipsky, Michael, and Marc A. Thibodeau. 1985. *Food in the Warehouses, Hunger in the Streets: A Report on the Temporary Emergency Food Assistance Program*. Cambridge: Massachusetts Institute of Technology, Department of Political Science.

———. 1988. Feeding the Hungry with Surplus Commodities. *Political Science Quarterly* 103: 223–44.

McDonald, Maurice. 1977. *Food, Stamps, and Income Maintenance*. New York: Academic.

Office of Analysis and Evaluation, Food and Nutrition Service, U.S. Department of Agriculture. 1987. *The Food Stamp Quality Control System*. Washington, DC: USDA.

Paarlberg, Don. 1980. *Farm and Food Policy: Issues of the 1980s*. Lincoln: University of Nebraska Press.

Panel on Quality Control of Family Assistance Programs, Committee on National Statistics, Commission on Behavioral and Social Sciences and Education. *Rethinking Quality Control: A New System for the Food Stamp Program*. Washington, DC: National Academy of Sciences.

Physician Task Force on Hunger. 1986. Increasing Hunger and Declining Help: Barriers to Participation in the Food Stamp Program. Cambridge, MA: Harvard University School of Public Health.

Public Voice for Food and Health Policy. 1989. Trends in Food Stamp Participation in the 1980s. *Rural Nutrition and Health Update* 2 (November).

Thibodeau, Marc A. 1985. Food as a Political Resource: The Cases of Chicago and Detroit. Master's thesis, Massachusetts Institute of Technology, Cambridge.

U.S. Conference of Mayors. 1983a. *Hunger in American Cities*. U.S. Conference of Mayors.

———. 1983b. *Responses to Urban Hunger*. U.S. Conference of Mayors.

Weekly Compilation of Presidential Documents. 1981. Cheese Inventory of the Commodity Credit Corporation. 17 (52).

Chronic Disease and Disadvantage:
The New Politics of HIV Infection

Daniel M. Fox

Abstract. HIV infection is now perceived as the end stage of a chronic disease that is spreading most rapidly among blacks and Hispanics. The politics of the HIV epidemic in the 1980s were dominated by four interacting factors: fear and fascination; who had the disease and to whom it seemed to be spreading; the endemic problems of United States social policy; and the impact on policy of advances in scientific knowledge. This paper analyzes the political history of each of these factors and describes the dominant policies of the federal government and the states regarding HIV in the areas of surveillance, prevention, research, and financing. Four uncertainties will have a profound influence on the future politics of the HIV epidemic: how the states and the federal government will address the general problems of paying for the care of people with chronic diseases and providing access to care for the uninsured and the underinsured; the number and distribution of the sexual behaviors that transmit infection with HIV and the effectiveness of policies to persuade people to modify these behaviors; precisely who uses addictive drugs and the effectiveness of measures to change their behavior; and the natural history of the virus.

A decade after AIDS emerged in the United States, most of the people who made health policy perceived it as a stage, at present the end stage, of a chronic disease that was spreading most rapidly among the disadvantaged, especially among blacks and Hispanics. This perception is the latest, and certainly not the last, chapter in a story that has changed repeatedly since 1981. As the story has changed, so has the debate about proper policy. This paper describes the politics of making policy for preventing the disease and caring for those who acquire it, among them some of the poorest people in this country.

The politics of AIDS to 1989

The brief political history of the epidemic has been dominated by four interacting factors: fear and fascination; who has the disease and to whom it seems to be spreading; the endemic problems of our social policy; and the impact on policy of advances in scientific knowledge. These factors created the political context for the current perception of AIDS as a chronic disease that is increasingly a burden for the disadvantaged and, as a result, for all of us.

AIDS, more accurately if ponderously called HIV infection and related diseases, has been a public issue out of proportion to its cost or mortality relative to such other contemporary afflictions as cancer, alcoholism, and automobile injuries. The standard, and probably accurate, interpretation for the high public salience of the epidemic—especially as revealed in coverage by the media—is fascination and fear: fascination with a disease that kills celebrities and those with homosexual lifestyles; fear of transmission through blood transfusion or sexual intercourse (Colby and Cook 1989). Moreover, as the incidence of the infection spread among urban blacks and Hispanics, fear of HIV intensified white people's dread of random aggression by darker-skinned males.

The public salience of the epidemic is also a result of longstanding problems of social policy in the United States. We lack consensus, nationally and in most of the states, about policy for public sex education and what (and how much) to do about drug addiction. Our employment-based private health insurance is least comprehensive in providing outpatient and long-term care and prescription drugs, which are growing costs of treating HIV infection. Medicaid eligibility and coverage varies widely among the states, leaving many persons who have HIV infection without effective entitlement to care. Moreover, states and local governments have enormous financial and political problems in serving as the health care payers of last resort.

These problems of social policy were exacerbated by both the politics of the 1980s and the epidemic of HIV infection. When the first cases of the syndrome to be called AIDS were reported in 1981, cost containment had become the priority of public policy for health financing, both for employers and for the insurance industry. A new national administration was determined to reduce federal domestic spending, including funds to assist the states in providing health care and social services to the poor. By the mid-1980s, when Congress and many of the states took new initiatives in health policy, AIDS was already a financial burden for several states, especially New York, New Jersey, California, and Florida, and was an emerging problem in most others (Fox 1988). Each new case represented a burden of about $100,000 in direct costs (Fox and Thomas 1989). As the number of cases increased among blacks and Hispanics—and as the number grew among women and children—these costs became a heavier burden on state and local governments. By 1989, perhaps half the costs of caring for persons with HIV infection had been paid by state and local governments—through their share of Medicaid, by insurance pools and indigent care programs, and by operating subsidies to public hospitals and clinics (Andrulis et al. 1989).

Attention to HIV infection in politics and social policy increased in 1989 for two reasons. The first reason was the rapid spread of infection and disease among members of disadvantaged minorities. Moreover, the incidence of infection with the virus among blacks and Hispanics was growing faster as a result of a newly observed linkage of crack, sex, and venereal disease. This new source of infection augmented to an ominous but unmeasurable extent its diffusion by needle sharing, by intravenous drug addicts having unprotected sex, and by women with the virus having children.

The second reason for increased concern was a new consensus among many health professionals and people who made policy that HIV infection must now be considered a chronic disease. From 1981 to the summer of 1989, the consensual view of the epidemic adopted the historical model of plagues. In this model, AIDS was analogous to the Black Death, yellow fever, smallpox, or polio. These diseases had emerged suddenly and unexpectedly, caused great devastation and, in time, receded for natural reasons or were vanquished by advances in prevention or treatment. Most proponents of the plague model insisted that AIDS would not recede soon. It was spreading around the world and had a long and imperfectly understood incubation period between infection and the appearance of symptoms. But many experts also argued, using the plague analogy, that AIDS required an emergency policy response because it was both an unusual and an unusually severe affliction. And many hoped that, as had happened a generation ago with polio and more recently with smallpox, heavy investment in research and in public health administration would contain or even eliminate the disease (Fee and Fox 1989).

The first challenge to the plague model of policy for the HIV epidemic derived from politics and policy analysis rather than from medical science and its applications. The challenge came from people who were absorbed with the problems of financing the epidemic. From the point of view of insurance executives, state Medicaid officials, and legislators addressing problems of the uninsured and hospital deficits, AIDS resembled a chronic disease that was compressed into a period of less than two years. Like other chronic diseases, AIDS was characterized by relatively brief acute episodes requiring hospitalization and longer periods when patients could be cared for in nursing facilities or at home. Like persons with other chronic diseases, persons with AIDS needed considerable social support, either from friends and families or from public agencies (Fox, Day, and Klein 1989). Unlike most people with expensive chronic diseases, however, most people with AIDS were not eligible for Medicare, either because they were under 65 or because they did not live long enough to become eligible for Social Security Disability Insurance (Fox and Thomas 1989).

This financially driven analogy to chronic disease was unpopular until the summer of 1989. Many advocates for persons with AIDS, especially gays, feared that defining the syndrome as a chronic infectious disease would lead to its "normalization." If AIDS became just another killer chronic disease, it would cease to evoke fear and fascination and, therefore, cease to have as large a claim on public attention and funds. Some scientists attacked the chronic disease model as defeatist. A few others, notably William Haseltine of Harvard, endorsed it (Haseltine 1989). Critics insisted that a disease that was spread by sex and drugs could not be considered simply another chronic disease.[1]

The chronic disease model became central to policy as a result of two clinical trials sponsored by the National Institutes of Health, one terminated in the spring and the other in the summer of 1989. The first trial justified the use of aerosolized pentamidine for persons who had had an episode of the most common complication of HIV infection, pneumocystis pneumonia. The other validated the use of AZT to postpone the onset of symptoms of disease secondary to HIV in certain patients. Both drugs resembled cancer chemotherapy more than the romantically misnamed "magic bullets" that cured many infectious diseases of bacterial origin, or the vaccines against major infections. Like cancer chemotherapy, the anti-HIV drugs inhibited the progress of disease, but did not prevent or cure it.

The new drug treatments created a new imperative and a new burden for policy. The imperative was that for the first time since the beginning of the epidemic persons who had engaged in risky behavior had a powerful incentive to be tested and, if infected, to receive prophylactic treatment. The burden was that treatment would be more expensive—but nobody could predict precisely how much more expensive, because it was based on new drugs. Moreover, the new drugs made the duration and course of the disease considerably more uncertain than before.

By the late summer of 1989 physicians and an increasing number of people who made health policy were describing HIV as the cause of a chronic illness with a long and lengthening course between infection and death. New diagrams that experts used to describe the disease to audiences of health and policy professionals exemplified the new perception of HIV infection. Throughout the 1980s, medical scientists had drawn an iceberg, with only the tip susceptible to treatment, to depict the disease; they now offered a timeline intersected by numerous and increasing opportunities for intervention (Cotton 1989).

While this shift of perception was occurring, the incidence and prevalence of HIV infection was increasing disproportionately among the disadvantaged. HIV infection and its consequences were, therefore, becoming a problem of American policy and politics as they affect minorities and the poor. AIDS had been normalized, but in a somewhat different way than advocates for according it higher priority had expected. The response to the disease was now part of the normal fragmentation and frustration created by our health policy

---

1. Personal communication with A. Brandt, 1989.

and disproportionately shared by the 40–50 million Americans who lacked minimal health insurance coverage and by the health and policy professionals who addressed their needs.

Perceiving HIV infection as a problem of the disadvantaged

The HIV epidemic offers elegant proof of the proposition that statistics contribute to but do not drive public policy. In the early 1980s, when most media attention and most advocacy for policy focused on AIDS as a disease of homosexuals, hemophiliacs, and recipients of transfused blood, overwhelming statistical evidence revealed that the epidemic was a disproportionately serious problem for blacks and Hispanics and that most of the people at risk of infection in these groups were of relatively low socioeconomic status. In 1982, the second year in which the federal Centers for Disease Control counted cases of AIDS, blacks and Hispanics comprised just under half of the males, almost 80 percent of the females, and almost two-thirds of the children diagnosed with the disease in the United States. In subsequent years the percentage of black and Hispanic men with AIDS ranged between 30 and 40 percent; the proportion of black and Hispanic women and children with AIDS was always considerably more than half (The Blue Sheet 1989a).

More important for gauging the impact of the disease on populations, and therefore on politics and policy, the number of cases per 100,000 population was always higher among blacks and Hispanics than among whites. By 1988 the cumulative total of cases per 100,000 was almost three and a half times higher among black men and two and a half times higher among Hispanic men than among whites. The rate among females was fourteen times higher among blacks and seven times higher among Hispanics. For children, the cumulative rates were four times as high among blacks and twice as high among Hispanics (Centers for Disease Control 1989).

There was, moreover, considerable evidence of undercounting of cases among blacks and Hispanics. In particular, intravenous drug users were recorded as dying at higher rates in these years from tuberculosis and other diseases which were, most likely, secondary to HIV infection, for which they had not been tested (The Blue Sheet 1989b).

By 1988, the rate of increase in reported cases was highest in cities with large black and Hispanic populations. This increase followed the pattern that had been observed earlier in the gay communities of San Francisco and New York and in other countries. As epidemiologists writing about Latin America described this pattern, once the virus was "introduced into a population, indigenous transmission soon became established and propelled the epidemic at an alarming rate" (Quinn et al. 1989). For example, in Newark, New Jersey, a predominantly black city, the rate of cases increased from 39 per 100,000 in the 12 months ending February 1988 to 56.5 a year later—a growth of 45 percent. In San Juan, Puerto Rico, an almost entirely Hispanic city, the rate of reported new cases increased by 78 percent to 66.5 per 100,000 in the same period. In San Francisco, in contrast, in a predominantly white population, new cases increased by only 12.7 percent in the same year. Published data reveal similar, though less dramatic, contrasts across the country (Centers for Disease Control 1989).

It is easier to describe than to account for the gradualness of the realization of the political and policy problems that result from the disproportionate impact of HIV infection on the disadvantaged. Several factors seem important in explaining what happened. One factor involves the politics of epidemiological evidence; the others involve the intersection of special interest politics with larger issues of social policy during the Reagan years.

The most important data about any epidemic, indeed about any problem, for most public officials and health professionals are the number and political influence of the people clamoring for scarce resources in a particular fiscal year. For the first eight years in which cases of AIDS were counted, the largest number of cases occurred among white males. The numbers of women and children—among whom the disadvantaged were an overwhelming majority— remained relatively low for most of the 1980s; the cumulative number of cases only reached 1,000 among women in 1986, and 500 among children in 1989. Prudent political professionals logically accorded priority to financing care for white males.

The second most important data about any problem for health professionals and public officials project its consequences into the practical future. The practical future for most elected officials is the year before and, sometimes, the year after the next election. For officials in the executive branch of state or local government, the practical future is the fiscal year after the one for which agencies prepared their most recent budget request. Most health professionals, especially those who treat patients or manage hospitals, have even shorter practical futures. They are trying to get through a day, a week, a few months, or a fiscal year. For both public officials and health professionals, projections of the incidence and demography of HIV infection three to five years into the future were ominous but not a problem for the practical future.

Official projections of the future number and demography of cases of AIDS had three other characteristics that reduced their political salience: they have been controversial; they are based on statistical reasoning rather than on field research; and most projections have not been targeted to particular jurisdictions.

Much of the controversy has been unavoidable. It is a result of ignorance about people's sexual behavior and drug habits, of congressional and White House opposition to or reluctance about asking people to describe these activities to interviewers paid with government funds, and of disputes among social scientists and biostatisticians about the accuracy of survey questions on matters about which many people are inclined to be evasive or dishonest. Moreover, strong opposition to mandatory testing for HIV or to reporting the names of people who test positive has come from civil libertarians, ethicists, gay advocates, and health professionals. These people have feared that mandates would, contrary to intent, persuade many people at high risk to avoid testing from fear of punishment or discrimination (Bayer 1989).

As a result of this controversy, projections of future cases of HIV-related disease have been based on statistical reasoning according to competing methods. When experts disagree about the future—even when, as in projections of the number of people with HIV infection, the range of their disagreement is narrower than their area of agreement—prudent public officials are highly motivated to temporize.

An even better reason for officials to temporize was the absence of credible projections for specific political jurisdictions. By 1989, only the cities and states with the highest number of cases had adapted any of the competing methods of projection for local use. Moreover, both AIDS activists and their adversaries frequently challenged the accuracy of these numbers. Credible and frightening data about the impact of HIV on minority communities came mainly from New York and New Jersey, states that are not normally regarded by people in other jurisdictions as harbingers of their social problems. Most states had relatively few cases of diagnosed AIDS—half had counted 200 or fewer through the first half of 1989—and hence no political incentive to sponsor local projections of controversial data.

The general condition of social policy and special interest politics reinforced the willingness of public officials to interpret data in ways that made it possible for them to avoid stark confrontation with the steady increase in AIDS cases among the disadvantaged throughout the country. There was little sympathy for expanding social programs in Washington or the states during the first Reagan administration. What sympathy existed was directed mainly at poor children, at working-age adults whose health insurance lapsed when they lost their jobs or whose employers were too marginal to purchase insurance, at people with disabilities who became ineligible for Social Security Disability Insurance as a result of new administrative procedures, and at the elderly who could not pay the catastrophic costs of illness or of long-term care. State officials were preoccupied in these years with policies to reduce the rate of increase in hospital costs in order to address competing pressures for new programs in health care, environmental regulation, welfare, and housing.

This picture of social policy in the 1980s is deliberately overdrawn. There were still many advocates for more health care for the disadvantaged. The people who managed health services that were traditionally aimed at black and Hispanic populations—clinics, health centers, hospitals, drug treatment programs—continued to lobby vigorously and effectively. Hospital leaders, alarmed at the growing cost of care for the poor and by the unwillingness of private insurance executives (themselves pressed by employers to reduce costs) to maintain traditional cross-subsidies, clamored for public funds to relieve their deficits. State government proposals to curtail Medicaid benefits or eligibility for coverage were often effectively opposed by associations of health professionals concerned about their earnings.

Nevertheless, for the first few years of the HIV epidemic, the states with the highest number of cases—especially New York and California—assumed that they would receive little additional assistance from the federal government and that most expenditures for AIDS, especially for testing, treatment, and support services, would be made as the result of state budgetary politics. In the politics of AIDS in New York state and California in the early and middle 1980s, doing it yourself meant taking action mainly in response to pressures from white gays and from the health professionals who treated them. Special interest politics reinforced the way public officials had chosen to interpret the epidemiological data.

Two special interests were involved: gays and blacks. Gay leaders in New York City and San Francisco built effective coalitions that leveraged funds for programs to prevent HIV infection, offer anonymous testing, and provide services for people with symptoms of disease. The coalitions led by gays were not opposed to helping poor blacks and Hispanics. Many of the service programs they established (notably the Gay Men's Health Crisis in New York City) provided considerable assistance to the disadvantaged. But they had other priorities: to promote safe sex among gays and—as both a goal and a shrewd political tactic—among white heterosexuals, and to provide better health and social services to people with the disease, the majority of whom were still white and gay. Understandably, too, they wanted to help gays who were also black or Hispanic, many of whom were not economically poor, but most of whom were discriminated against by other blacks and Hispanics.

At the same time, many black leaders were unwilling to advocate that special attention or funds be given to the problem of HIV infection in their communities. Their refusal to become advocates for particular interventions to prevent the spread of infection, especially for the interventions urged by most white public health leaders, reinforced the disproportionate attention to HIV among white gays.

The reluctance of many black leaders to become special interest lobbyists on behalf of those infected with HIV had complicated, overlapping causes. In a recent essay, Harlan Dalton of the Yale Law School explains the political and cultural logic of reticence about AIDS among African-Americans. He isolates five "overlapping factors": wariness about acknowledging "our association with AIDS so long as the larger society seems bent on blaming us as a race for its origin and initial spread"; the "suspicion and distrust many of us feel whenever whites express a sudden interest in our well-being"; the "pathology of our own homophobia"; the "uniquely problematic relationship we as a community have to the phenomenon of drug abuse"; and "difficulty transcending the deep resentment we feel at being dictated to once again" (Dalton 1989).

Some of these factors also influenced the behavior of Hispanic leaders in the early years of the epidemic. Most accounts (in the press and by other politicians) stress homophobia as the most important reason for the unwillingness of these leaders to be perceived as special interest advocates for AIDS sufferers.

The politics of the epidemic changed quickly late in 1989, especially in the cities and states with the highest incidence of cases. The priorities in fighting a plague are learning where it came from, taking emergency action to protect endangered communities, and creating crash programs to experiment with vaccines and potential cures. The priorities of managing a chronic disease are different. These priorities are familiar to everyone who has followed the recent history of lung cancer, heart disease, stroke, or renal disease. Preventing new cases of chronic disease is a difficult and expensive process. Fear and education are effective, but there is no consensus about how much of each to use and what techniques have which effects on particular people. Treatment is expensive and arduous. Moreover, effective treatment means incremental improvement, not cure (Fox 1989). Plagues are fought; chronic diseases are managed.

By the end of 1989 the coalition demanding more resources for HIV infection had changed and its membership remained in flux. Prominent blacks were becoming part of the HIV lobby—for example, joining leadership coalitions in several cities and nationally. Dalton, for example, was appointed by Congress to the new National AIDS Commission. Advocates for spending more to prevent and treat HIV were included in the constituency for President Bush's drug abuse initiative. Black and Hispanic advocates for persons with HIV infection (and for minority physicians) were demanding new roles in the politics of research as NIH awarded the first contracts for community-based clinical trials intended to increase the enrollment of disadvantaged people. The increasing cost of care for people who were chronically ill with HIV infection was bringing new pressures on federal and state officials to pay for prescription drugs and increase access to outpatient and long-term care services for members of minority communities. In addition, these new political alignments were occurring when, for the first time in almost two decades, many leaders of state government, industry, and labor were eager to rethink our customary arrangements for financing health care, including the care of the poor.

Policies for HIV infection among the disadvantaged

The coalition on behalf of people with the chronic disease of HIV infection will probably obtain incremental changes in existing policies. More fanciful scenarios will be proposed, but there is little reason to expect that fundamental changes in our national health policies, or in those of the states, will be more than talk for the next several years. It is therefore useful to describe what the dominant policies regarding HIV are, how they affect the increasing proportion of infected people who are disadvantaged, and what incremental changes seem feasible. Four areas of policy are important: surveillance, prevention, research, and financing.

Surveillance is likely to become more aggressive, and less responsive to the concerns of civil libertarians and advocates for minority groups. Surveillance means both counting the number of people with infection and at various stages of the disease and projecting those numbers into the future. Several major assumptions of surveillance policy for the epidemic had changed by the end of 1989. Before then, the incentive to be tested for individuals whose behavior placed them at risk of HIV infection was to learn whether and how to avoid infecting others, or if they were fortunate, to protect themselves. Now that there was a prophylactic therapy, individuals who might be infected had reason to be tested, not just for antibodies to the virus but also for the level of T4 cells in their immune system. Moreover, there was a better case than before for creating registries of the names of infected people, in order to offer them additional testing and treatment as new interventions became available. Such testing and treatment might be particularly beneficial for disadvantaged people who are or were addicted to drugs and for their children.

There are now new incentives to learn more about the changing levels of infection in particular populations in order to estimate more precisely both near-term costs and the effectiveness of various techniques to prevent infection. Accuracy in counting cases remains an important goal of policy, but for more hopeful reasons than measuring the demographics of the epidemic and projecting costs. Moreover, the risks to persons from breaches of confidentiality will have to be weighed against the benefits of counseling people to enter treatment. Even informed consent for testing might be exchanged for therapeutic benefit in some states; for instance, by routine testing of all newborns for HIV infection, similar to the testing now conducted in every state for phenylketonuria.

Similarly, prevention policy is expanding to include measures to delay the onset of disease symptoms as well as to reduce the number of people who acquire or transmit the virus. Preventing the onset of symptoms requires persuading people to have their T4 cells tested regularly and to receive chemotherapy. Policymakers and advocates for communities in which many poor people live will have to decide whether to create new programs of outreach and treatment or to couple preventive treatment for HIV with existing programs of primary care and of treatment for addiction.

Policies to prevent people from acquiring or transmitting the virus are also likely to change as a result of the perception that HIV is a chronic disease that is uncommonly prevalent among members of minority groups. Many prominent black and Hispanic leaders who have opposed needle exchange programs, for example, may be increasingly interested in assessing the results of research on their effectiveness in Europe and the United States. The impressive evidence that programs to persuade addicts to change their needle-using behavior reinforce each other and do not discourage addicts from entering drug treatment programs (Des Jarlais 1989) may become politically salient if leaders of minority communities believe that they have more responsibility for choosing among alternative policies.

Research policy has also been affected by the new perception that HIV infection is a chronic illness that occurs disproportionately among disadvantaged people, especially minorities. The new NIH program of community-based trials is one example of change. Another, perhaps more important, change is the creation of faster-track drug approval processes by NIH and FDA. Faster tracks were a response to advocacy by gay leaders and their allies in the research community. FDA policy might change more rapidly if more black and Hispanic leaders join coalitions pressing for changes in it. Finally, the unprecedented outcry by both advocates and public officials about the pricing policies of drug companies (especially of Burroughs Wellcome, which makes AZT) has stimulated industry accommodation and may lead to changes in policy, as the cost of treating HIV infection and the public share of the cost increases.

Financing treatment for persons with HIV infection will be the most difficult area of policy in which to effect changes. Treating HIV infection is expensive and will become more so when more people are tested earlier and repeatedly and receive treatment over a longer period of time. It is too soon to conjecture whether newly approved treatments will decrease hospital cost for each case, the most expensive component of care. More important is the context in which political discussion about financing treatment of HIV infection occurs. Most state officials continue to assume that the states will be the payers of last resort, even for treatment with newly approved drugs. Legislative leaders report that they are under increasing pressure from advocates for people with other diseases who worry that persons with HIV infection are getting preferential treatment (Fox 1990). There are orphan drugs, but politically, there are no orphan diseases.

In late 1989, public health officials in several states with the highest incidence of HIV disease began to mobilize support for larger and broader federal subsidies, especially for prescription drugs. They argued that new drug treatments made the cost of treatment prohibitive, especially because the incidence of HIV disease is growing most rapidly among people without private health insurance. In the summer of 1990 Congress authorized the expenditure of $2.9 billion over five years for planning and services in the cities and states with the highest incidence of HIV infection. The act was named for Ryan

White, the Indiana teenager whose exclusion from school had attracted national media attention in 1985, and who had died in the spring of 1990. But naming the act for White did not disguise the fact that it provided services mainly for the disadvantaged in a tough budget year that was also an election year for the Congress. In the budget compromise of 1990, the Ryan White Act received only a token appropriation.

The most important impediment to successful political advocacy for additional federal financing of treatment for HIV disease may be that it is one among many areas of inadequacy in health care financing and organization. Only a few political leaders, even in the states with the most cases of AIDS, are willing to risk being accused of fixing the AIDS problem while they neglect others. Many state political leaders and representatives of health care interest groups who say that they would join a coalition to promote federal legislation to address access to care for the uninsured, the underinsured, and the poor are refusing to support legislation that is limited to HIV (ibid.).

Moreover, few states are likely to legislate comprehensive solutions to the problems of financing treatment for HIV infection. Not surprisingly, in the epidemic to date, state financing policies have been a result of past and present health politics, particularly the politics of Medicaid, rather than of the number of cases of disease. In the HIV epidemic, as for most other illnesses, equality of access to health care is not yet an attainable entitlement. For Americans of working age and their children, where they live and for whom they work continue to be the major determinant of what care they can have and how it will be financed.

There have been three stages in state responses to the epidemic, each stage a result of the interaction of politics with the incidence of disease. In the first stage, a state relies on its existing policies for financing health care and regulating the institutions that provide it. Toward the end of the first stage, states earmark appropriations to pay for care of persons with AIDS. New York was the first to earmark funds. By 1986 states that earmarked funds included, among others, California, New Jersey, New Mexico, and Ohio.

In the second stage, states make deliberate decisions about how to adapt their Medicaid policies and regulations and often initiate state-only programs to address some of the problems of financing and organizing care for persons with HIV-related diseases. The most frequently implemented policies concerned "waivers," a ruling by the Health Care Financing Administration (HCFA) that a state may make a particular mix of Medicaid services available to some but not all beneficiaries on the condition that the proposed services will not add to federal costs. By the end of 1988, HCFA had granted waivers to six states (California, Hawaii, New Jersey, New Mexico, Ohio, and South Carolina) to reimburse care for persons with AIDS in homes or community facilities as a substitute for acute hospital care. Several other states had waivers pending. Moreover, other states—Illinois and North Carolina, for example—

financed treatment for persons with AIDS as part of a broader grant of waiver authority (for the aged and disabled) from HCFA.

Other states decided not to seek a waiver. Several did not apply for a waiver in order to avoid potential costs or because officials believe that the problem of financing care for HIV-related disease is not yet pressing. In other states— New York and Michigan, for example—the decision not to seek a waiver had other sources. In New York, officials decided that Medicaid was already covering "almost everything that was waiverable." In Michigan, in addition to a "rich service package," officials believe that waivers are difficult to administer (ibid.).

In 1989, 27 states appropriated funds for patient care for persons with HIV-related diseases in addition to their Medicaid programs. Eighteen of these states also made appropriations for support services. Most of these funds subsidized inpatient care for people with low incomes, but they were also used for hospices, outpatient clinics, case management services, and, in ten states, to purchase and administer AZT (Rowe and Keintz 1989).

In the third stage (reached to date only in California, New York, and to a lesser extent in Michigan and New Jersey), states, in collaboration with other payers and institutions, adopted policies for organizing and financing care that go beyond the population eligible for Medicaid services. In New York, for example, the AIDS Treatment Center program begun in 1986 mandated enhanced reimbursement to hospitals from all payers for inpatient care and for case management of ambulatory and long-term care. New York also provides enhanced reimbursement rates in long-term care facilities. In California, the Department of Health Services funded 26 pilot projects to provide some health and attendant care, subsidized hospice services, and has established a new institutional category, a "licensed health care facility for persons with AIDS." In the summer and fall of 1989, New Jersey established a new program, apparently the first in the country, of "assessment centers," to encourage early detection of infection, regular testing for the level of T4 cells, and the use of AZT to retard the onset of symptoms. The state provided the start-up costs for this program; Medicaid and private insurers covered most of the ongoing costs (Fox 1990).

By 1990, three states had explicitly addressed the problem of financing care for persons with HIV infection as part of the larger problem of access for the uninsured and the underinsured. A 1989 Michigan law required the Department of Social Services to "identify potential Medicaid recipients who test HIV-positive and pay their insurance premiums so that they can maintain their health insurance policies." The state of Washington implemented a similar HIV/AIDS insurance continuation program. California had a continuation program, but only for persons who were already eligible for Medicaid. Officials in all three states acknowledge that these programs are pilots for addressing other chronic diseases that lead to financial impoverishment and have high public costs (ibid.). Efforts to legislate a similar program in New York failed in 1990, mainly as a result of opposition from an aroused insurance industry that was eager to avoid what would be certain losses.

Because it is new, spreads so rapidly, and is expensive to treat, HIV infection reveals more clearly than most diseases do the flaws in the collection of laws and customs we call health policy. But recognizing flaws creates both problems and opportunities. There is no lack of clever solutions to the problems of health policy in the United States. There is, however, no politically effective coalition at the present time, either nationally or in any of the states, that is willing to pay the price of legislating any of the more fundamental solutions.

The future of policy for HIV and the disadvantaged

Four uncertainties will have a profound influence on the politics of the HIV epidemic. One, discussed above, is how the states and the federal government will address the general problems of paying for the care of people with chronic diseases and of providing access to care for the uninsured and the underinsured. The price of the epidemic of HIV infection will surely increase, whether new strategies to finance treatment are specific to this epidemic or address the fundamental problems of health policy in the United States. What is uncertain, however, is the total price and the politics of paying it.

The other three uncertainties arise at the intersection of politics and policy with biology and human behavior. The first is uncertainty about the natural history of the virus—if and how it will mutate, and how it will respond to efforts by scientists to produce vaccines to inhibit its infectivity and drugs to reduce or prevent its effects.

The second is uncertainty about the number and distribution of the sexual behaviors that transmit infection with HIV and about the effectiveness of various policies to persuade people to modify these behaviors. There is little evidence about the number, distribution, race, ethnicity, and socioeconomic class of homosexuals, of bisexuals, and of heterosexual people who practice unprotected anal intercourse. Moreover, there is little research-based knowledge about the relative effectiveness of various methods of inducing fear and prudence in changing people's sexual behaviors.

The third area of uncertainty concerns precisely who uses addictive drugs and the effectiveness of measures to change their behavior. Estimates of the number of people who use intravenous drugs are mainly conjectures based on extrapolation from the number of people who seek treatment. Moreover, little is known about the linkage of crack, heightened sexual activity, venereal disease, and HIV infection. There is impressionistic evidence that drug-using behavior among more affluent people is linked to HIV infection in areas as diverse as the suburbs of New York (Thomas and Fox 1989) and rural Georgia.

Evidence about the effectiveness of programs to persuade drug users to change their needle-using and sexual practices has, to date, been more persuasive to advocates than to political leaders.

These uncertainties, taken together, make impossible any predictions, or even very many recommendations, about future policies. Numerous alternative scenarios are being debated. In 1990, the authors of most of these scenarios assumed that the epidemic would become increasingly expensive to treat as a result of advances in therapeutics and that it would continue to have a disproportionate impact on blacks and Hispanics. Thus most scenarios assumed that persons with HIV disease would make increasing claims on scarce public funds but that it is unlikely that a powerful coalition of political leaders who have white, relatively affluent constituencies would be eager to grant these claims. At the end of 1990, most political leaders seemed to agree that the public attitude (and that of most of their colleagues) toward HIV infection had become "massive apathy," as one powerful state legislator said.

Scenarios are inevitably extrapolated from current events. As recently as 1987, for example, a few serious scenarists were conjecturing a rapid spread of HIV infection among affluent white heterosexuals. By 1989, such a scenario was regarded as alarmist. In 1986 and 1987 most scenarios assumed that AIDS was a disease with a relatively swift and terrible course that would, for the near future, not be treatable. By 1989, most health professionals talked about AIDS as the end stage of a chronic disease of uncertain course that could be modified by chemical therapies. Any scenario is likely to be wrong.

For almost a decade, however, HIV infection has dramatized the dilemmas of health policy in the United States. HIV disease is an expensive disease to manage, but our policies distribute most of the resources for managing expensive diseases through Medicare and Medicaid payments for long-term care for the elderly. Prevention is the most cost-effective intervention, but we know very little about the effectiveness of different strategies and have no routine way to pay for implementing them. We spend an unusually large proportion of our national income on health care, but increasing numbers of people are dependent on the inadequate care that is provided by state and local government as payers of last resort. We generously finance biomedical science, but the results of that effort do not translate quickly into measures that reduce the incidence and pain of disease.

In sum, the epidemic of HIV infection continues to reveal what many people already know about health policy in the United States. By doing so, the epidemic clarifies the difference between knowledge and power, and between concern, even compassion, and effective political will.

References

Andrulis, D. P., U. B. Weslowski, and L. S. Gage. 1989. The 1987 U.S. Hospital AIDS Survey. *Journal of the American Medical Association* 262: 784–94.

104   Daniel M. Fox

Bayer, R. 1989. *Private Acts, Social Consequences*. New York: The Free Press.
The Blue Sheet. 1989a. AIDS Cases in the United States, 1982–88. 22 March, p. 8.
———. 1989b. CDC AIDS Surveillance Data Omits One-Third of Current Cases. 28 June, p. 3.
Centers for Disease Control. 1989. *HIV AIDS Surveillance*. Atlanta: CDC.
Colby, D. C., and T. E. Cook. 1989. The Mass-Mediated Epidemic: AIDS on the Nightly Network News, 1981–1985. Paper presented at a meeting of the International Communication Association, May.
Cotton, D. 1989. AIDS/HIV Infection: A Medical Update. Presentation to a workshop on "The Use of Health Services Research to Develop Policies Addressing the AIDS/HIV Epidemic," sponsored by the U.S. Public Health Service in Timberline, OR.
Dalton, H. 1989. AIDS in Blackface. *Daedalus* 118: 205–28.
Des Jarlais, D. 1989. Approaches to Reduce High-Risk Behavior in the Drug Abuse Population. Presentation to a workshop on "The Use of Health Services Research to Develop Policies Addressing the AIDS/HIV Epidemic," sponsored by the U.S. Public Health Service in Timberline, OR.
Fee, E., and D. M. Fox. 1989. The Contemporary Historiography of AIDS. *Journal of Social History* 23: 303–14.
Fox, D. M. 1988. AIDS and the American Health Polity: The History and Prospects of a Crisis of Authority. In *AIDS: The Burdens of History*, ed. E. Fee and D. M. Fox. Berkeley: University of California Press.
———. 1989. Policy and Epidemiology: Financing Health Services for the Chronically Ill and Disabled, 1930–1990. *Milbank Quarterly* 67 (supp. 2, pt. 2): 257–87.
———. 1990. Financing Health Care for Persons with HIV Infection: Guidelines for State Action. *American Journal of Law and Medicine* 16: 223–47.
Fox, D. M., P. Day, and R. Klein. 1989. The Power of Professionalism: Policies for AIDS in Britain, Sweden and the United States. *Daedalus* 118: 93–112.
Fox, D. M., and E. H. Thomas. 1989. The Cost of AIDS: Exaggeration, Entitlement and Economics. In *AIDS and the American Health Care System*, ed. L. Gostin. New Haven: Yale University Press.
Haseltine, W. 1989. Prospects for the Medical Control of the AIDS Epidemic. *Daedalus* 118: 23–46.
Quinn, T. C., F. R. K. Zacarias, and R. K. St. John. 1989. AIDS in the Americas: An Emerging Health Crisis. *New England Journal of Medicine* 320: 1005–7.
Rowe, M., and R. Keintz. 1989. Natural Survey of State Spending for AIDS. *Intergovernmental AIDS Reports* 2: 1–10.
Thomas, E., and D. M. Fox. 1989. AIDS on Long Island: The Regional History of an Epidemic, 1981–1988. *Long Island Historical Journal* 1: 92–112.

Health Care Policy Issues in
the Drug Abuser Treatment Field

William E. McAuliffe and Kathleen Ackerman

Abstract. Recent decades have seen profound changes in the nature and extent of drug abuse and in government and industry responses to it. Any discussion of policy, however, should take into account the fact that the needs of the public sector are very different from those of the private sector. Legalizing drugs would not solve the problems of either sector—the argument for it is based on mistaken assumptions, and the execution and management of such a policy would be impracticable. In the public sector, the main policy goals should be to define and fund the levels of care, lengths of stay, and quality of care that are needed to combat heroin and cocaine epidemics and the spread of AIDS among intravenous drug users. In the private sector, on the other hand, the main goal should be to control costs by limiting the growth of the burgeoning private drug treatment industry and by rationalizing levels of care, lengths of stay, and quality of care for middle-class and middle-aged drug users.

As we enter the 1990s, drug abuse is once again at the top of the list of society's problems. The recent epidemic of crack use and resulting violent crimes have alarmed the public. Adding to their concern is the spread of AIDS among intravenous drug addicts and the realization that addicts are the disease's main bridge to the general population (*Focus* 1989). President George Bush has launched yet another war on drugs. Frustration has led some local officials to employ methods that may impinge on civil rights (Graham 1989), while others have called for the legalization of drugs of abuse.

Several other major changes have occurred in the last two decades, which should affect the development of health policy for drug abuse. Those changes include the spread of serious drug abuse into middle-class and middle-aged populations, the growth of a large for-profit chemical dependency industry, research that has resulted in a new theory of what constitutes addiction and how to treat it, and methodological breakthroughs in epidemiology and the

Grants from the National Institute on Drug Abuse (DA05271 and DA04418) and from the Division of Substance Abuse, Rhode Island, supported work on this article.

evaluation of drug abuse treatments. This essay will examine the implications of each of these changes for health policy and the drug abuser in the 1990s.

An important starting point is to distinguish between policies that apply to the public and private sectors (see Gerstein and Harwood 1990). Although the issues overlap, there is enough difference between the two sectors to result in what might appear to be contradictory policy recommendations. The major policy problem in the public sector is the chronic inadequacy of funding to meet societal needs, whereas the major problem in the private sector is control of expanding costs to third-party payers. Confusion could result if policy discussions failed to consider the differing needs of each sector. For example, drug abuse professionals who have toiled for years in the public sector often become angry when they read of the need for cost-containment regulations in the field. Planners, insurers, and regulators, however, are faced with rapidly rising costs in the private sector that threaten to undermine recent breakthroughs in third-party coverage of substance abuse problems (Freudenheim 1990). Certificate-of-need regulations designed to control costs in the private sector may inadvertently have an even greater impact on development of badly needed public-sector services. We will therefore analyze the sectors separately, attempting to point out how and why they differ.

We will focus on health care policy, planning, and regulatory issues concerning nonmedical drug abuse. We will not include tobacco, caffeine, or alcohol in our discussion, because many policy issues involving these substances differ from those regarding controlled drugs. Our essay is based on a needs assessment and treatment plan that William E. McAuliffe and his coworkers prepared recently for Rhode Island (McAuliffe, Breer, White, et al. 1988; McAuliffe, Breer, Ahmdifar, and Spino 1991) and on McAuliffe's current studies of cocaine addiction and AIDS prevention.

Legalization of drugs of abuse

"Legalization" of controlled drugs is the latest drug policy fad. It is a criminal justice concept rather than a health policy, but could have major implications for health policy were it adopted. Recent calls for drug legalization, mostly from a mixed group of frustrated lawyers and judges, conservative economists, urban politicians, and persons long associated with liberal attitudes towards drugs (Nyhan 1990; McConnell 1991), react to the record levels of urban homicides and shootings (Associated Press 1990) caused by gangs and small-time dealers competing for profits from cocaine distribution. Addressing only one aspect of the drug problem, legalization nevertheless appeals to a frightened public's desire for a quick, painless (inexpensive) solution. At the other extreme are proposals for questionable uses of force, including the proposal to use the armed forces against South American drug cartels, and New Hampshire's decision to have troopers test driver's licenses for cocaine because it is a "quick, easy, and unobtrusive way to obtain evidence in drug cases" (Hohler 1990a).

The legalization argument.   The proposal to legalize controlled drugs is premised on the assumption that the current war on drugs is primarily punitive, has been adequately tried, and obviously has not worked in the past (Nadelmann 1989). The war on drugs, legalization proponents argue, will be just as ineffectual as previous wars against drugs. The core rationale for legalization is that removing the legal restrictions to access to drugs would "get the money out of drugs" and thereby eliminate black market drug trafficking and the high prices of drugs and violent turf wars associated with it without causing an unacceptable increase in the extent of drug use, addiction, and associated health and social problems (McConnell 1991). Drug abuse would be controlled by shifting criminal justice funds to treatment and prevention programs.

So far, however, legalization is only a general approach or catchphrase (Nadelmann 1989), and not a policy. Public debates over legalization have produced few details on how the concept would be implemented, especially in the case of highly dangerous drugs like heroin and cocaine, the drugs that produce most of the violence and crime filling the newspapers. When pressed for details, legalization advocates talk of marijuana decriminalization (McConnell 1991; Nadelmann 1989), but are unprepared to venture specifics about the drugs that are causing all the problems. At a recent legalization conference, Andrew Weil, a well-known legalization proponent, was quoted as saying, "I really would like to see some serious work done in the next few years to come up with a whole range of options for what legalization might look like, very concrete images of what this would mean, whether it would mean going to a pharmacy or some kind of panel licensed to buy certain things. We should be very specific and concrete" (McConnell 1991). The persistence of the legalization idea probably depends on this very lack of detail, for it is unlikely that radical drug legalization would achieve widespread support.

American drug policy.   Despite the arguments by legalization proponents or the rhetoric of politicians, our drug-control policies over the last twenty years have been neither full-fledged nor concerned exclusively with criminal justice solutions. Previously declared "wars" on drugs were in actuality not wars at all. Proposing harsher penalties, such as death for drug dealers, makes for good headlines and campaign rhetoric, but it has little impact on drug abuse. Although drug-related arrests and the total number of persons in prison rose steadily in the 1980s (Jackson 1989), and funding for criminal justice approaches has outstripped money for treatment (Gerstein and Harwood 1990), the criminal justice system has been playing catch up. Drug addicts have usually outnumbered narcotics police by as much as 1,000 to 1. That ratio might make sense for policing the general public, but hardly for a population that contains a high percentage of habitual criminals.

Consider, for example, the drug "war" in Boston. In 1985 (before the crack epidemic arrived) the city assigned 20 narcotics police to combat an estimated 14,000 heroin addicts (Murphy 1990). It is anyone's guess how many additional persons there were who used heroin occasionally or who were addicted to other drugs. Heroin addicts accounted for only half of the persons receiving drug treatment in Massachusetts (McAuliffe et al. 1986). It is also relevant that the Boston metropolitan area has an estimated 450,000 students attending college, and college students have high rates of drug use when compared to the general population (McAuliffe, Breer, White, et al. 1988). A survey of University of Wisconsin–Stout students found that 4 percent reported addiction to illicit drugs (Cook 1987). If that percentage were true for Boston, the drug control unit would have to deal with an additional 18,000 addicted college students. The Boston drug control unit increased threefold by 1990, but even that number of police can hardly be expected to fight an effective campaign against abusers of heroin and crack, in addition to college student drug abusers, during the peak of a drug epidemic. With so few drug control police available, one can go to certain street corners in American cities such as Boston and find hundreds of heroin addicts dealing and buying drugs at any time of the day.

There is already evidence that promises made when the current war on drugs was declared are not being fulfilled. A Boston newspaper recently reported that embittered local police said, "Because of massive fiscal problems at the state and local level, the commitment by politicians to wage the fight has fallen short of their fiery rhetoric of bygone days" (Kennedy 1991).

Added to the inadequacy of police resources is the neglect in the rest of the criminal justice system. It is well known that jails are overcrowded, by as much as a factor of seven in some Massachusetts jails. Chronic drug offenders, who account for a significant proportion of the prisoner population, are often released early merely to relieve crowding, and some states, such as Connecticut, have also cut costs by eliminating parole departments which could supervise the offenders who received early releases (Hohler 1990b).

Despite the rhetoric of previous drug wars, American drug policy has long included a significant treatment and prevention effort. Judges rarely mete out the harsh penalties that politicians see as their main answer to the public's concerns about drugs. Tough-sounding legislators grab headlines and infuriate civil libertarians by passing death penalties for major drug dealing, but in fact no one has ever been executed as a result of dealing drugs, no matter how large the amount. Only a small percentage of drug arrests actually result in incarceration. In practice, judges would much rather divert drug cases to treatment, especially to drug-free programs such as therapeutic communities. Of course, declining funding for treatment has reduced this option to a significant degree.

Proponents of legalization almost never mention that quasi-legalization schemes have been implemented in this country and elsewhere for more than two decades. Methadone maintenance programs have legally distributed powerful opiate drugs to heroin addicts since the late 1960s. The only major pharmacological difference between methadone and heroin is the speed of the drug action. Methadone taken orally is as effective as heroin in controlling withdrawal symptoms, but is less pleasure-producing because it is a longer-acting drug and it has a much slower onset than injected heroin. (Oral administration also prevents most drug-related health problems.) Recently, many states have adopted "for-profit methadone maintenance." In these programs, heroin addicts pay out of pocket for methadone, and counseling services are often less emphasized. In some states public funds pay the program fees so that the drug is free to the client. Other states are experimenting with "medical maintenance" programs for long-term, well-functioning methadone clients. These programs charge modest prices (ten dollars or less) for a day's supply of methadone and do not require any form of therapy. The client merely picks up the drug from a pharmacist each day. The only other restriction that methadone maintenance places on the addict is that the dosage is relatively fixed, but it is often more than the equivalent amounts of heroin typically used on the streets. Having a stable dosage is important to avoid accidents or overdoses and to allow the client to live a relatively normal, productive life. There are also large numbers of addicted chronic pain patients who receive small daily doses of opiate medications from their personal physicians without anyone taking special note of it (McAuliffe 1982). It seems unlikely that any acceptable legalization policy would be much more than an expansion and slight liberalization of these programs.

Thus, American drug policy has always been lots of tough talk but relatively little action. Neither the criminal justice nor the treatment approaches have been adequately funded, except perhaps briefly when an epidemic pushes the problem to the top of society's list of social problems. The American approach has always included both treatment/prevention and criminal justice approaches. Included in the treatment component since the late 1960s has been a quasi-legalization scheme, even if it has not been called that. The greatest change over the last twenty years has been in the relative standing of the two. Whereas treatment and prevention received more federal funding than did criminal justice during the early 1970s, in the late 1970s the two were about equal, and in the 1980s criminal justice received two to three times as many federal dollars as did treatment/prevention (Gerstein and Harwood 1990).

Consequences of legalization.   What results could we expect if our society decided to deemphasize criminal justice measures radically while liberalizing access to drugs? Contrary to claims of legalization proponents, there is some evidence that previous wars against drugs that contained some restrictive policies have been effective. A prohibition of cocaine use in the United States was effective in the early 1900s (Musto 1989), and an epidemic of opiate addiction resulting from quasi-therapeutic uses (e.g., elixirs and patent medicines) was eliminated by narcotics laws. When the Nixon administration spent large sums to combat the heroin epidemic of the 1970s (*Journal of NIH Research* 1989: 28), the epidemic declined (Dupont and Greene 1973). The Japanese effectively contained an amphetamine epidemic following World War II by a series of restrictive measures (Tamura 1989). There is also evidence that recent efforts to tighten controls over prescription drugs have borne some fruit, with emergency room visits down by one-third since 1981 (Skorneck 1989), and that even this latest cocaine epidemic is tapering off (see below). Obviously, these policies have not prevented periodic epidemics, such as the present one, but it is hard to say that they have been totally without effect.

Since proponents of legalization typically support their position by pointing to the "failure" of Prohibition, it is important to consider carefully the difference between alcohol use in the 1920s and our current drug problem. Consumption of alcohol had much greater public support prior to the passing of the Volstead Act in 1919 than consumption of cocaine and heroin do today. There is nevertheless ample evidence that alcohol consumption declined substantially during Prohibition, even if related crime increased to unacceptable levels. Consumption of marijuana, which continues to be widely used by youth (one-third of high school students at last count) and whose adverse effects are more comparable to alcohol than to heroin or cocaine, lacks the cultural and religious legitimacy that alcohol consumption has enjoyed for centuries in American society. There is every reason to believe that the laws against nonmedical use of drugs of abuse are effective in constraining consumption, certainly more effectively than taxes and licensing requirements have proven to be in reducing the consumption of tobacco and alcohol.

Black markets.   Although the black markets and turf wars of Prohibition disappeared with repeal, experience with methadone maintenance suggests that it is far from certain that drug black markets would be easily eliminated. While current evidence suggests that the amount of street crime (e.g., burglaries or theft) committed by heroin addicts declines when they are maintained on methadone, the black market in heroin has persisted even at times when methadone treatment was abundant. If the economists favoring legalization are right, one would at least expect heroin to be cheap as a result of competition from the methadone programs that give opiate drugs away for free or for nominal fees. Since this expectation has not been borne out dramatically, if at all, one must question the assumptions that underpin the legalization argument.

Since the 1920s, Great Britain has distributed morphine, heroin, or methadone along with cocaine to addicts in injectable form by prescription for nominal fees (Schur 1962). This program eliminates many of the addicts' objections to the American methadone maintenance approach. The British system has not, however, eliminated the heroin-related crime problem or drug trafficking (McAuliffe 1980). The system was designed and worked effectively for iatrogenic addicts and addict health professionals; it broke down when American and Canadian heroin addicts migrated to London and nonmedical drug use became popular there. Many British addicts, especially youths and neophytes, then refused to take advantage of the legal drugs (Glatt et al. 1967), and many who received them also used black market drugs as supplements. A common pattern was for addicts to use their three-day drug allotment of legal drugs within a few minutes of leaving the clinic and then buy black market drugs until it was time for the next legal allotment (Glatt et al. 1967). Others sold all or part of their legal allotments to friends, thus creating a black market. Since the 1960s the number of addicts in Great Britain has grown fiftyfold, and the British have adopted steadily *more* restrictive policies as their heroin addiction problem has worsened.

Elimination of black markets would depend, no doubt, on how liberal the legalization policy would be. It seems unlikely that the American public could accept the open drug marketing to neophytes, the skid-row squalor, crime, overdose deaths, and high rates of AIDS found in some of the free drug zones in Europe. Consequently, until advocates of legalization make clear what they would do with regard to heroin and how they would avoid the problems the British and other Europeans have encountered, it is unclear what the legalization idea has new to offer even on the criminal justice front.

Health.   Perhaps the greatest concern about legalization is that the more radical the policy, the more likely it is to result in substantial increases in health problems. Our experience with Prohibition provides clear support for this prediction. While Prohibition failed to eliminate drinking altogether and produced a black market, it succeeded in reducing alcohol consumption by 30 to 50 percent. That led to a dramatic decline in both cirrhosis deaths and hospital admissions for alcohol-related psychosis (Moore 1990). With the legalization of commercial alcohol manufacture in 1933, alcohol consumption and related disease increased significantly.

This experience with controlling alcohol suggests that if use of heroin or cocaine were totally uncontrolled, many more Americans would use them and experience various side effects, including addiction. Although advocates of legalization hold that there are a relatively fixed number of persons who would use drugs such as heroin and cocaine even if they were made legal (Nadelmann 1989; McConnell 1991), the history of controlled drug abuse in this country suggests that the opposite is true (O'Donnell 1969; McAuliffe 1975). The number of users and abusers in the United States has increased enormously in the last twenty years, far beyond the levels that anyone would have predicted in the early 1960s and beyond levels in other countries. Our drug abuse problems of today, including the turf wars, are a direct result of that growth. At the beginning of this epidemic, defenders of liberalizing marijuana laws argued that its use by youth would not result in the use of more dangerous drugs such as heroin and cocaine. Unfortunately for our society, they were wrong, especially in the case of cocaine. Many people do not use drugs because doing so is dangerous and illegal, and because they are not subjected to the aggressive commercial marketing that could accompany more radical legalization plans. There is little reason to believe that under legalization the amount of heroin or cocaine consumption in the United States would remain unchanged. Users of "legalized" drugs would seek treatment for addiction just as Americans sought treatment for addiction to narcotics long before its use was controlled by law (Terry and Pellers 1928). It is likely that the demand for treatment would increase substantially.

If use of cocaine and heroin increases substantially, the frequency of drug overdose deaths, hepatitis B, AIDS, and other drug-related diseases is likely to increase sharply. Advocates of legalization often ignore this problem by generalizing from experiences with relatively less dangerous drugs, particularly tobacco, alcohol, and marijuana, to the most dangerous, cocaine and heroin. In the process they also seem to exaggerate the dangerousness of tobacco and alcohol while downplaying the dangerousness of controlled substances (Hadaway et al. 1991; Nadelmann 1989). Legalization proponents therefore imply that drugs such as heroin and cocaine can be controlled effectively with taxes and licensing in the same manner as we control tobacco and alcohol.

Our system of drug controls is based primarily on the fact that use of some drugs is riskier (by experimental and epidemiological evidence) than use of others. Historical factors also play a role. Although every drug has risks (e.g., even aspirin can produce an addiction if used enough), some have so few risks that they can be used without controls by the general public. Alcohol and tobacco are in that category. Other drugs that have greater risks have greater controls (e.g., require a prescription). Despite the great risks of some drugs, they may be prescribed for use under a physician's direction and in specified ways (e.g., no refills). Under very controlled conditions, even these drugs may have sought-after beneficial effects that cannot be obtained any other way, and the controls minimize the risks. Cocaine and morphine are in that category. Heroin is comparable to morphine but is not used for medical reasons in the United States primarily because it is so notorious as a drug of abuse, and there are many other opioid drugs that are equally effective.

Uncontrolled use of controlled drugs such as heroin and cocaine in a large, urban society such as ours would no doubt result in severe health problems, far worse than the health problems stemming from tobacco or alcohol use. Whereas long-term use of opiates is generally safe under a doctor's direction (e.g., methadone maintenance), uncontrolled use produces many overdose deaths, has severe neonatal effects, and increases the risk of associated diseases such as hepatitis and AIDS (Petitti and Coleman 1990). Legalization proponents (Nadelmann 1989; Hadaway et al. 1991) claim that restrictive drug laws cause these health problems, but uncontrolled use of heroin and cocaine is highly dangerous even when the drugs are obtained in pure form from a pharmacy and where drug controls are lax. For example, AIDS is spreading rapidly among addicts in England, Switzerland, and the Netherlands. Drug overdoses and injection-related infections such as hepatitis are as prevalent among heroin addicts in Great Britain as in the United States (Blumberg 1976).

Although alcohol and tobacco account for more deaths each year than do cocaine and heroin (Nyhan 1990), the consumption of alcohol and tobacco by millions of users is so much more extensive in both amount and years of use than the consumption of heroin and cocaine that the comparison is not meaningful. Most Americans (85 percent) have drunk alcohol at least once, and over 100 million people (53 percent of the population) say that they currently drink (National Institute on Drug Abuse 1990: 19). By comparison, only 7 percent of the general population of Rhode Island reported having ever tried cocaine (McAuliffe, Breer, et al. 1988); nationally, an estimate 10.7 percent had ever used cocaine in 1988, and only 1.5 percent had done so in the previous thirty days. The figures for heroin are probably one-tenth the size of those for cocaine. Six percent of the national sample had used marijuana in the previous month. Thus, a national sample of respondents in 1988 was nine times more likely to be currently using alcohol than cocaine, and about three hundred times more likely to be using alcohol than heroin. Consequently, if there are more people addicted to alcohol or tobacco than to controlled drugs, one should not declare to the public that alcohol is "the single most addictive drug" (*Parade Magazine* 1989) or that tobacco is "the most addicting of all drugs" (McConnell 1991).

Nor should one imply that alcohol or tobacco are as dangerous as controlled substances. Dose for dose, health problems are much less likely or less severe for alcohol or tobacco than for cocaine and heroin. Acute drug effects, such as overdose deaths, are unknown for tobacco and rare for alcohol. The number of emergency room visits for cocaine effects more than tripled between 1985 and 1987, and for the first time outnumbered those for every other controlled drug, including heroin, which was the leader in previous years (Drug Abuse Warning Network 1989; *NIDA Notes* 1988–89: 1). The visits for heroin, the next most frequent in 1989, were one-third those for cocaine. Heroin overdoses each year kill about 2 percent of heroin addicts. Even among controlled drugs there are large differences in the degree of danger. Marijuana use is far more extensive than that of either cocaine (by a factor of about three) or heroin (by a factor of about thirty), but in 1989 there were six times as many emergency room visits for cocaine and two times as many for heroin as for marijuana (National Institute on Drug Abuse 1990). Data from emergency rooms in Rhode Island for 1987, 1988, and 1989 show that there were eight times more visits related to alcohol than to cocaine—far fewer than one could expect if alcohol and cocaine were equally harmful (Hachadorian, Campbell, and Tellier undated [1987, 1988]; Campbell, Hachadorian, and Tellier 1990).

Recent evidence also indicates that we may have underestimated the role of controlled drugs in automobile accidents (Budd et al. 1989; Sweedler 1991). In a study of 182 fatal truck crashes, one-third of the drivers tested positive for drugs or alcohol. Marijuana use was as common as alcohol use (13 percent each), and cocaine use was not far behind (9 percent). Our own interviews with heroin addicts indicated that most had accidents as a result of the drug's intoxicating effects; it is frightening to contemplate how many automobile accidents would result if 53 percent of the population used heroin regularly.

Most of the health effects of tobacco are the result of years of use, but we are just beginning to learn what the comparable long-term effects of heavy cocaine smoking are. The acute diseases caused by repeated sniffing and injecting of cocaine are already well known, and there is a growing body of literature documenting the multiple adverse consequences of chronic cocaine smoking. AIDS will probably kill 25 to 50 percent of the intravenous addict population in the next ten years. That in no way diminishes the problems that alcohol and tobacco cause, but it would be highly misleading to assume that widespread cocaine and heroin use would be no more dangerous than current use of tobacco or alcohol. It is also quite likely that the increase in death and disease resulting from a drug policy as radical as legalization proponents seem to be suggesting would far outweigh the unacceptably large number of homicides and wounds resulting from the cocaine turf wars.

The demand for drugs.   There is one argument of the legalization lobby which is undeniable. A strategy to control drug use by reducing supply will have limited effect in the face of strong demand. The principal cause of the current drug problem is the American public's twenty-five-year tolerance of recreational drug use. In the mid-1960s, at a time of great economic prosperity, Americans were convinced that the harm of drug abuse had been exaggerated by government officials for their own narrow ends, and that drugs such as marijuana and LSD were beneficial and carried little risk of progression to drugs such as cocaine or heroin. The acceptance of cocaine and its subsequent rise to the second most popular drug were clearly the result of a similar change in perception. In a decade or two cocaine was transformed from being perceived by the public as a highly dangerous and potentially addictive drug to being seen as a harmless substance that was exciting and conferred status on its users. The fact that large parts of the public are still willing to consider the possibility of uncontrolled cocaine use demonstrates that they still do not fully accept or comprehend its inherent danger.

A critical part of the solution to this problem is therefore to convince the public that nonmedical drug use is too dangerous when seen in a long-term, societal perspective. Events since the 1960s have only slowly altered the public's beliefs. After many deaths (Len Bias's was especially important), treatment admissions for people addicted to cocaine (including well-known figures), and countless pictures of cocaine-addicted children left at hospitals, the public is beginning to believe that cocaine use is dangerous. In general, it has taken the experience of several decades of personal and collective experience to persuade a majority of the American public that the drug proselytizers of the 1960s were wrong. Our youth are finally becoming convinced of the adverse effects of drug use.

Many have erroneously concluded from this shift in attitude that the answer to the drug problem is not law enforcement but drug education in the schools (Lehigh 1990). History has shown, however, that educational messages delivered at school or through late-night public service announcements have a limited effect. Education has surely been tried—most school systems have had drug education in the curricula since the mid-1960s. Experimental studies have demonstrated that such programs have had very limited success even after years of trying. It is also obvious that drug education, like criminal justice efforts, has failed to halt the huge increase in drug use since the 1960s.

Drug education has too often floundered because at the same time our youth were getting a very different message from a much more powerful source. While teachers were warning about drug use, the media—magazines, television, and motion pictures—were advertising exotic drug effects and the glamour of drug use through stories of drug fads and pictures of drug use by trendsetters in the arts, sports, and centers of wealth. The many magazine cover stories on cocaine in the mid-seventies and subsequent newspaper accounts and television portrayals all contributed to the change in attitude. Pleasurable drug effects, improved sex, and exclusive clubs and social scenes were described in detail. Discussions of the possible risks of excessive use were inevitably included at the end of the article or TV show. Young people easily convinced themselves that they could enjoy the immediate pleasures of drugs that were described without falling victim to any adverse consequences. A big-city fad quickly became a national obsession, and the demand for South American supplies spread into every American community. Even now, stories of the problems that drugs cause inevitably include pictures of someone sniffing cocaine with a rolled one-hundred-dollar bill. Although there is some research on learning how to use media to prevent drug use, we should give some thought to preventing it by not inadvertently promoting it in the first place.

There has never been a concerted intellectual effort to answer drug-use proponents. Even the legalization issue has not been pursued as energetically by knowledgeable government spokesmen and scholars who oppose it as by those who favor it. The rise in drug abuse and its many problems resulted most of all from a change in public attitudes, especially among youth. That change occurred when proponents of drug use were victorious in the debate over whether or not drugs were truly harmful. When a new drug became popular, scientists were careful to note that there was insufficient evidence to be sure that it was harmful. Proponents were quick to conclude that it was therefore harmless. From the late 1960s, these national debates over drugs were given a great deal of airtime. Drug-use proselytizers actively contradicted the message of drug educators, thereby giving encouragement to experience-seeking youth. Debates over legalization have also received an inordinate amount of media attention, even though no bills have been entered and no legislature is seriously about to adopt it. Legalizing drugs makes for a tantalizing story, whatever its merits as a national policy. But such stories and debates may have profound effects on the public, especially our youth. Once the public believed that drugs could be used without harm, all government programs, whether criminal justice or prevention and treatment, were powerless to prevent the resulting epidemic from running its course. We clearly need to pay more attention to these debates, for misinformation and misinterpretation that either exaggerate or underestimate the risks of nonmedical drug use are counterproductive.

Adoption of some form of legalization would thus send the wrong message to the public at a time when attitudes have started to change and the consumption of drugs by youth has been diminishing gradually. This decline in drug use has continued for almost a decade and has now reached record lows (*NIDA Notes* 1989a). Despite recent headlines, there is good reason to believe that the current epidemic is diminishing. This is no time to take desperate action, either to the left or to the right.

The likelihood of legalization is becoming ever more remote. The latest surveys indicate that drugs have slipped from the very top of the list of urban concerns after three years (Leavitt 1991), and drug czar Bennett has stepped down, declaring that the drug war is behind us. A recent news report on the proceedings of a major conference on legalization stated that the conference's messages were, "The 15 minutes of fame and flurry a year or so ago about legalization of illicit drugs in the United States has faded, and proponents have to realize it is going to be a long, hard slog if there is ever to be success" (McConnell 1991).

Even if legalization were implemented, society would still have to confront the issue of how to pay for and regulate the delivery of addiction treatment. Since legalization is improbable and certainly not a panacea for our drug woes, the remainder of this article will attend to more familiar and perhaps more mundane policy issues that nonetheless are likely to be implemented and that others have not addressed at length.

Policy issues in the public sector

In the past, health policy in the drug abuse field seemed out of step with most of the health care field. Drug abuse was a disease confined primarily to poor, inner-city youths and young adults, and services for this population were supported by direct federal or state government allocations. There was little third-party coverage for drug treatment services, and therefore issues that preoccupied the rest of health care, such as cost containment and quality of care, were not major topics in the drug treatment field. As with other health services for the poor, such as treatment for the chronically mentally ill, low levels of government funding effectively constrained costs. Staff received low salaries, facilities were often poorly maintained, and services were effectively rationed by having no public programs in some areas and long waiting lists in those areas that had programs. For many years the major health care policy concerns in the public sector were limited resources and the limits on quality imposed by the lack of staff training and qualifications. The policy picture has changed primarily in response to epidemics of heroin addiction, AIDS, and cocaine abuse.

The heroin epidemic.   The first major development in drug treatment policy resulted from an epidemic of heroin addiction. In the 1950s nonmedical drug abuse (primarily heroin addiction) was worrisome, but still a minor problem for most Americans. Addiction to heroin (or related opiates) had been declining since 1920, and the addict population was quite small by today's standards. Whereas there were an estimated 60,000 heroin addicts in the entire country during the decade of the 1950s, today there are an estimated 40,000 addicts in Baltimore alone, and New York City probably has ten times that many. The treatment system for the entire U.S. consisted of two public service hospitals, a few detoxification beds in state psychiatric hospitals, and occasional private sanitaria for therapeutic addicts and addicted self-medicating health professionals. Since two out of three heroin addicts were unemployed (McAuliffe and Gordon 1974) and the rest were underemployed, employers did not have to provide for workers suffering from drug abuse. Alcohol abuse was the only major substance abuse problem in the workplace, and there was little third-party coverage even for alcohol treatment.

The situation began to change in the 1960s and early 1970s. A major heroin epidemic occurred in our inner cities. Drug abuse was high on the national agenda when the Nixon administration responded (radically at the time) by funding methadone maintenance and other forms of drug treatment on a large scale, helping states plan rational treatment systems, primarily for treating heroin addiction, and establishing the National Institute on Drug Abuse (NIDA) in 1974 to lead the effort. The services were funded primarily directly by NIDA and states (Gerstein and Harwood 1990: 213), and were targeted to lower-income populations.

Funding for drug abuse services then declined in real dollars through the 1970s and mid-1980s (Schuster 1990; Gerstein and Harwood 1990) as the prevalence of general nonmedical drug use and abuse apparently grew steadily

(McAuliffe, Breer, White, et al. 1988). The heroin addiction problem seemed to abate briefly in the 1970s, but after a period of excess treatment capacity, the demand for services grew again. Despite this renewed growth in heroin addiction, governments were unwilling to devote significant new resources to it. Peaking in the early 1970s, NIDA funds (nominal dollar amounts) for community drug treatment services remained unchanged during the remainder of the 1970s despite substantial inflation. The Reagan administration switched from direct federal funding to state block grants in 1982, and in the process substantially reduced the amount of federal funds devoted to drug treatment (Gerstein and Harwood 1990). The states failed to make up the difference (Gerstein and Harwood 1990: 212), and all the states that we have worked with, including Rhode Island, Massachusetts, Maryland, and Connecticut, have had significant shortages of services for treating their heroin addict populations.

Since there are many people who continue to have doubts about the idea of distributing methadone to addicts, it is not surprising that some localities withdrew public funding for methadone entirely. While for-profit methadone programs helped fill the void, many heroin addicts left treatment (Anglin et al. 1989). Observers believe that our public-sector drug treatment system is far worse now than it was in the 1970s (*Journal of NIH Research* 1989). In an assessment of treatment needs for Massachusetts, McAuliffe (1986) discovered significant shortages of methadone services, and in the Rhode Island needs assessment (McAuliffe, Breer, White, et al. 1988), we recommended that the amount of publicly funded treatment slots be doubled immediately.

Thus, one of the roots of the current drug problem appears to be the unwillingness of government to maintain its commitment to provide adequate drug treatment services to the poor, especially when there is an increase in demand. The signs that an expansion of services was needed were obvious (long waiting lists at virtually every methadone program, detoxification facility, and therapeutic community, and no programs at all in many areas that had experienced an influx of addicts since the 1970s). Unlike many other health problems that afflict the poor, there was no automatic mechanism for responding to increased demand for drug treatment, because drug abuse services were not widely reimbursed by Medicaid. Moreover, after the peak of the heroin epidemic had passed, there was little talk of increases in government allocations for drug treatment until the AIDS and crack epidemics caught the public's eye in 1986 and 1987. By contrast, there has been a steady increase throughout the period in the federal funds allocated for criminal justice approaches to the drug problem.

The AIDS epidemic.   The AIDS epidemic is certain to cause many problems for the public-sector drug abuser treatment system, but for now it has had the positive effect of bringing the shortage of services to the public's attention.

It is clear that intravenous drug users are the primary vector in the spread of the AIDS epidemic to the general population. As a result, rates of HIV infection among some minority populations have grown to frightening proportions already (St. Louis et al. 1990). Fear of AIDS is one of the prime reasons for the current growth in federal funding for treatment and outreach services and for the willingness of states to fund more drug detoxification and methadone maintenance services, including expansion of drug treatment services reimbursed by Medicaid. For example, in Massachusetts the new administration has stated that AIDS prevention will be one of the few service areas that will not be cut back.

The AIDS epidemic among intravenous (IV) drug users has naturally become a critical health policy topic in the drug field. The combination of weak leadership among government officials, especially during the Reagan years, and the increasing availability of federal and state funds for local programming has occasioned many local struggles. Furthermore, no network of IV/AIDS organizations has taken the reins of power, as happened in the gay community. Each of the contending groups (primarily AIDS organizations and drug treatment providers, but also church officials, homeless shelter officials, community activists, federal grant and demonstration project recipients, medical researchers, and state health officials) has its own perspective on what should be done and who should lead the effort. A large part of the confusion is that no one is sure whether IV/AIDS is primarily an AIDS problem or a drug use problem. AIDS organizations rarely have the expertise to serve the AIDS prevention and support needs of intravenous drug users. Also, the policies (regarding testing, methods of behavior change, and the mix of support services) and staffing patterns of many AIDS organizations were developed for a largely gay client population and may not be optimal for intravenous drug users. Many local drug treatment programs have viewed AIDS funding as a way of meeting long-standing resource shortages, but street outreach, prevention, and coping with the problems of the terminally ill have rarely been the mainstay of these agencies. This leadership vacuum makes it difficult to reach a consensus on policy, utilize resources effectively, or mobilize the overall community.

Even at the federal level, there is now some question about which agencies should direct the fight against AIDS in the addict community. The Centers for Disease Control were slow to act initially, apparently because they lacked the relevant expertise, but now they appear eager to take the leadership role that initially defaulted to NIDA. NIDA has developed substantial expertise in investigating epidemiological, prevention, and treatment questions with this population. Adequate needs assessment and planning for AIDS prevention require such expertise. Virtually all drug abuse researchers have looked to NIDA for funding and guidance over the years, and NIDA has maintained a relationship with drug abuse prevention and treatment providers through its research and demonstration programs. Although AIDS prevention among intravenous drug users has some similarities with AIDS prevention among other groups (e.g., testing and AIDS education), it consists primarily of drug treatment and street corner outreach. Moreover, public health professionals have historically paid more attention to prevention of tobacco and alcohol abuse than to treatment of intravenous drug abuse. Recent federal policy has nevertheless transferred the authority for IV/AIDS prevention services from NIDA to the Centers for Disease Control, leaving NIDA to play primarily a research role. NIDA's national network of IV/AIDS outreach programs is in the process of being dismantled just three years after being formed. It could take the CDC years to develop comparable capabilities.

To date, the major policy issues surrounding AIDS have involved the political dilemma of how to fight the disease without encouraging drug abuse or sexual misconduct. The general public and many political leaders, including conservative forces in affected communities and the treatment community, would like to believe that the AIDS epidemic among intravenous drug users can be stopped by education, moral persuasion, and more traditional forms of treatment (especially drug-free forms). Health officials, researchers, and AIDS activists doubt that these approaches will do the job. They have advocated needle exchange programs, free distribution of methadone from vans (based on the Dutch model), and distribution of bleach bottles and condoms by outreach workers.

Our research in Baltimore (McAuliffe, Breer, and Doering 1989) and current work in Massachusetts suggest that the latter group is probably closer to being right. There is no clear-cut evidence on the extent to which the mass of public information has slowed the spread of HIV among intravenous drug users. It seems quite likely that addicts have responded to some degree, but in one of our study cities there was a seroconversion rate in excess of 10 percent in the last year. Education alone offers little hope for slowing the rate further, since addicts already know about AIDS and how they can reduce their risk of getting it. The Baltimore study found that outreach workers providing only AIDS education and referrals to treatment were not sufficient to change significantly the high-risk behaviors in this population.

It is also clear that providing traditional drug treatment on demand is not the sole answer. Although there are shortages of treatment resources and manpower that must be eliminated, states have been unable to fill these gaps quickly enough to stem the rapidly growing epidemic. In Massachusetts, shortages of drug treatment still exist almost five years after officials became aware of the situation. In addition to fiscal constraints, state officials have had great difficulty finding communities that would allow siting of methadone programs, even when the communities themselves had a large untreated addict population with high rates of HIV. There is also no system for giving infected addicts priority when there are openings in existing methadone treatment programs, which would help prevent the spread of HIV to other addicts, the majority of whom are still not infected.

Although treatment offers an important measure of protection against becoming infected, it is not foolproof. Our Baltimore study showed that many intravenous drug users who are in treatment were still engaging in risky behaviors (sharing needles and having unprotected sex) (see also Chu et al. 1989). Most who are not already in treatment do not want to enter traditional forms of treatment (McAuliffe, Breer, White, et al. 1988), and many of us fear that these drug users are the ones who are most at risk of infection. The federal government recently suggested reducing some of its regulations regarding ancillary services that methadone maintenance clients must accept, but this idea was quickly withdrawn when it was met with skepticism both from methadone treatment providers and from segments of the community that have historically worried about the misuse of methadone maintenance for political ends. When these two groups join forces with conservative community elements, health officials have a hard time sustaining any liberalization of treatment policy.

Distributing bleach bottles, making confidential HIV testing easily available, and developing more accessible nontraditional treatment forms are probably the most effective and politically acceptable methods of preventing the spread of HIV among intravenous drug users. There is growing evidence that many addicts have added bleaching to their needle-cleaning practices, but as a rule addicts are not bleaching as often as they should. Unfortunately, states are currently prohibited from using federal block grant funds for bleach distribution. Some addicts might also benefit from having easier access to clean needles, but evidence from European sources suggests that needle exchange— like treatment and education—is only partially effective in preventing the spread of AIDS. Although needle exchange proposals have caused the greatest political uproar in this field, resistance to needle distribution has enhanced the appeal of less radical approaches, such as bleach distribution and increases in methadone treatment services.

It is likely that voluntary HIV testing is a more important means of controlling the epidemic in the intravenous drug user population than many experts recognize. HIV testing in drug treatment programs has raised issues in the drug field as it has in the gay community. Anti-testing AIDS activists have raised concerns about the possible negative impact of HIV testing on persons early in recovery (Verdone 1989), while many addicts have shown a desire to be tested, especially when testing is made readily available (Weddington and Brown 1988). As evidence mounts that early detection and treatment offers substantial advantages to the infected person, and that testing is an important tool in preventing the spread of the disease by HIV-positive individuals, resistance to HIV testing is declining in the field (Rhame and Maki 1989; Casadonte et al. 1990; Robertson et al. 1988; McKeganey 1990).

Our current research suggests that many addicts who are not interested in traditional forms of treatment would utilize nontraditional forms, such as Narcotics Anonymous and addict drop-in centers, or will utilize telephone crisis counseling or informal counseling from outreach workers they see on the streets, in shelters, or through home visits. Our recent experience suggests that many of those who use the nontraditional treatment modes will eventually accept more traditional services.

No doubt the most serious AIDS issues will surface when large numbers of HIV-infected intravenous drug users become sick and need increasing amounts of medical care, housing, and support services. Our research has found an overall infection rate of 25 percent among addicts recruited from the street corners of three medium-sized Massachusetts cities, and a rate of 50 percent among fifty black and Hispanic addicts recruited from one of the cities. It will not be long before these infected addicts seek expensive forms of medical care and support services, and many infected intravenous drug users in our study are already homeless.

The cocaine epidemic.   The public's perception of the drug problem today is clearly linked to the widespread use of cocaine. Never before in our history have so many Americans used a drug as dangerous as cocaine. Cocaine, especially when used intravenously or smoked, is as addictive as heroin (Hasin et al. 1988). Whereas fewer than 1 to 2 percent of the general population has ever tried heroin, cocaine is now second only to marijuana in frequency of use. Seven percent of the Rhode Island population has tried cocaine (McAuliffe, Breer, White, et al. 1988), and 48 percent of third- and fourth-year medical students in Massachusetts have done so (McAuliffe, Rohman, et al. 1986). Between 66 percent and 80 percent of the drugs seized by police in Massachusetts are cocaine. In many states, such as Rhode Island, cocaine currently accounts for more requests for drug abuse treatment than any other illicit drug, including heroin. We have grown accustomed to news of drug-induced train wrecks, plane crashes, and fatal accidents in the workplace and on our highways (Sweedler 1991).

Among lower socioeconomic groups the cocaine problem has taken the form of a crack cocaine epidemic. Crack is a form of cocaine that can be easily smoked by "freebasing." Because crack is smoked rather than sniffed, it is absorbed more quickly into the body (comparable to intravenous injection) and is therefore more dangerous with respect to risk of overdose and onset of addiction. There is, however, no fundamental difference between the drug effects of crack and those of any other form of cocaine. Many long-term heroin addicts have converted to crack cocaine or, in some cases, a combination of cocaine and heroin. Cocaine abuse has also become a major problem for ex–heroin addicts on methadone maintenance.

It is noteworthy that the headlines have focused on the short-term effects of crack, including shootings, increased emergency room visits, and the health problems of crack-using mothers and their children. The wave of street murders caused by gangs and traffickers scrambling to profit from the crack market contrasts sharply with previous heroin-related crime waves, which primarily involved property crime to obtain money for a heroin dependence. If the crack epidemic is similar to other drug epidemics (Hunt 1974), other long-term effects of chronic cocaine use, such as a rise in the number of crack addicts seeking drug treatment or needing medical care for lung and heart disease, may continue to surface for several years past the peak of use. Street crime and other short-term effects of crack use may, however, serve as early warning signs that lead the government to fund more treatment slots now, thereby reducing the likelihood of a major treatment crisis in future years.

At present, there are no standard treatment modalities for cocaine addiction, and the chronic lack of resources has made it difficult for the public sector to respond to the crack epidemic with respect to the number of treatment slots and needed changes in the content of care. Since much of the public sector drug treatment system was designed primarily to handle heroin addiction, many facilities (e.g., methadone maintenance programs and short-term methadone detoxification units) are not equipped to treat the crack addict. While methadone is useful for treating opiate addiction, we have no comparable drug for treating persons addicted to crack. Long-term drug-free residential facilities (therapeutic communities) are suitable for treating crack addiction, and in many facilities cocaine addicts have overtaken heroin addicts as the most frequent patient type. Outpatient drug-free treatment and aftercare modalities have received little attention as cocaine treatments up to now, but our research suggests that they may be the treatment of choice for many working- and lower-middle-class cocaine addicts. It is also clear that self-help meetings, such as Cocaine Anonymous, can serve lower-income addict populations.

Policy, planning, and regulation in the 1990s.   The prime needs in the public sector are to fill current gaps in service, develop mechanisms that will insure long-term adequate funding, develop cocaine-specific treatments, and attend to the previously ignored issues of levels of care, length of stay, and quality of care. Although increased federal funds are on their way to the states to help fill current treatment gaps, any remaining shortages can be closed in several ways. Partial copayment strategies and for-profit methadone counseling services fitted to the specific needs of clients can be expanded steadily, especially for working- and lower-middle-class addicts, for those with mild psychiatric problems, and for those who have been in methadone treatment for a year or more and are employed. Methadone maintenance without counseling ("medical maintenance") is so inexpensive that many addicts will be able to afford it. Expansion of Medicaid reimbursement for the full range of services would help meet current needs and would insure the long-term financial stability that is currently missing (see below). Facilitation of self-help programs is another strategy that is often overlooked. One of our current projects has provided meeting space that has increased the number of Narcotics and Cocaine Anonymous meetings in Cambridge, Massachusetts, by a factor of five or more. Between three and four hundred addicts attend these "beginners" meetings every week.

The field needs to develop long-term funding mechanisms that will upgrade the quality of services and avoid the yo-yo effect of funding that responds only to epidemics that have gotten out of hand. Since neither heroin addicts nor the people who care for them have political clout, drug abuse services should be tied to services that enjoy a wider base of support. Like most social services and psychiatric services, drug treatment for the poor has suffered from public disinterest and lack of commitment, even in periods of economic prosperity. Massachusetts had waiting lists for methadone maintenance while it was expanding services in many other areas. When the so-called Massachusetts economic miracle ended, there was already a severe shortage of services for cocaine addicts and intravenous drug users. The obvious answer is that substance abuse services for the poor should be funded by the same insurance mechanisms that cover the rest of medical care for the poor. Although no one wants to add to an overburdened health care bill, there is little justification for excluding substance abuse as a health care problem among the poor and especially the homeless.

The public drug treatment system needs to be modernized if it is to respond effectively to the crack epidemic. Treatment research on crack addiction is also needed, since most of the early research on treatment of cocaine addiction has been conducted on middle-class, white populations. Retraining heroin-oriented staff to deal with cocaine addiction is another important item for the agenda as we enter the 1990s.

Levels of care.   The drug treatment field has generally not devoted adequate attention to providing the full range of levels of care. Heroin addiction in inner cities has been treated with highly supportive therapies, including short-term detoxification, long-term residential care (therapeutic communities), and outpatient methadone maintenance. Aftercare was poorly developed by most modalities, with the possible exception of therapeutic communities. Outside the inner city, where there are only small concentrations of opiate addicts, most addicts are treated through generic outpatient drug-free counseling following hospital detoxification. Outpatient drug-free treatment usually involved one hour a week of individual or group counseling. As a result, opiate addicts either remained in highly supportive programs beyond the point of necessity, which wasted resources, or did not receive adequate levels of support upon discharge from brief but intensive hospital or residential treatment.

Drug treatment experts have long questioned the cost-effectiveness of detoxification services, and consequently most states have devoted few resources to detoxification. Addicts are known to enter detoxification as a mere respite from addiction without any intention of seeking long-term recovery. Relapse rates are high (e.g., 15 to 20 readmissions is not unusual for some clients), and inpatient detoxification facilities tend to be medically oriented and therefore expensive (as much as ten times the cost of outpatient drug-free services).

Animal models of addiction have led to a reconceptualization of the fundamental nature of the disease and its diagnosis and treatment (McAuliffe, Albert, et al. 1990–91). Whereas addiction was once regarded as primarily a physiological disorder, most scientists now view it as primarily a result of drug conditioning, where the key biological mechanisms are the reward centers of the brain. Physiological detoxification (as distinct from cessation) as a cure for physical dependence is now viewed as only the beginning of some forms of drug treatment, and it is not even an essential feature of other forms of addiction treatment, such as treatment of crack addiction. Although this new model of addiction has had a major impact on drug abuse research and diagnosis already, only recently has it begun to have an impact on drug treatment. This conditioning theory of addiction emphasizes the need for a sufficiently long period of outpatient treatment of gradually declining intensity that allows for the controlled extinction of drug-related stimulus-response connections. "Relapse prevention" is a recently developed outpatient drug abuse treatment that exemplifies this new understanding of addiction and its treatment. Other recent innovations, including "day care," "evening care," and "recovery houses," provide intermediate levels of care that were previously mostly absent from the drug treatment field. Regulatory decisions about levels of care and lengths of stay will no doubt be affected directly by this new theory.

The AIDS epidemic has, however, brought many new actors into the drug policy arena, and they bring with them the old physical theory of addiction for which detoxification is the logical solution. Enthusiasm for acupuncture detoxification among AIDS activists (Pittman 1991) also appears to stem from an emphasis on the importance of detoxification. Since the general public also believes that detoxification is tantamount to cure, political pressure has produced an increase in detoxification services in the short run. In the private sector cost inflation has led to a serious effort to examine the need for expensive forms of treatment such as detoxification and the value of less expensive forms of intermediate levels of care, but it is unclear whether there will be a parallel mandate in the public sector.

Lengths of stay. Publicly funded treatment modalities do not have the resources to provide adequate treatment to all lower-income addicts who want it or to provide adequate adjunctive services for many who are in treatment. But neither have they always used the resources they do have in the most efficient way. Methadone maintenance has a tradition of lifetime treatment (based on an unsubstantiated metabolic theory of its efficacy), and clients with ten to twenty years of maintenance treatment are not unusual. A minimal standard level of care is required for all methadone maintenance treatment, no matter how long-term, although some relaxation of procedures is possible if a client has made good progress for a number of years. We have questioned the wisdom of having an unlimited length of stay and a fixed level of care (McAuliffe, Breer, White, et al. 1988). The current system often discourages addicts who wish to detoxify voluntarily and requires an addict to accept as much as twenty years of group and individual counseling (the most expensive components of methadone maintenance treatment) as a condition for receiving methadone. We believe that clients should not be required to accept unwanted services, especially when other clients cannot receive the more intensive services they need and want, and persons on waiting lists are receiving no services at all.

In Rhode Island, methadone providers were quite upset by the idea that existing resources could be used more effectively from the standpoint of the overall system if clients were discharged sooner to provide openings for the many clients who were on the waiting list (McAuliffe, Breer, White, et al. 1988). From a clinician's standpoint, it is usually better for the individual client to remain in care as long as he or she wishes, but any additional improvement in the client's long-term outcome is likely to be smaller than the improvement in outcome for the person on the waiting list who would otherwise receive no care at all. This issue came to the attention of the regional methadone providers group, which quickly mobilized pressure from the entire region. When the federal government recently suggested that regulations would be modified to relax the counseling requirements for methadone clients to allow for expansion of the number of clients per program, many long-time providers condemned the change as countertherapeutic. Unfortunately, to date there have been no experimental studies that have investigated the cost-effectiveness of varying lengths of stay; there are studies in progress that are investigating the cost-effectiveness of different levels of counseling services in methadone maintenance. Clearly, the perspectives of providers and planners can be quite different on such matters, and some objective data would be useful.

Long-term residential treatment facilities, known as "therapeutic communities," also have a tradition of substantial lengths of stay, usually more than a year and sometimes as long as two and a half years. Since such treatment is much more expensive ($10,000 per year) than outpatient treatments (about $2,500 per year), therapeutic communities have begun to offer shorter courses of residential treatment. Continued investigation of new models of this form of treatment is an important priority for the new decade.

For outpatient drug-free counseling, the typical length-of-stay standard for state-funded treatment facilities is as long as a patient has an issue to discuss. Although the actual number of months in outpatient drug-free counseling is usually relatively small, that criterion for determining the length of stay should give one an idea of the sharp differences between the drug field and the result of health care on such matters. Development of behavioral criteria for completion of various treatment levels could be a useful goal in the present decade.

Regulators are sure to encounter substantial provider resistance to shortening these traditional lengths of stay in the public sector, and they must be alert to the unique features of the system and its client population when developing regulatory mechanisms. Historically, the field has been primarily concerned with how to get and keep clients *in* treatment, not how to get them out as soon as possible. Professionals have long fought to establish that substance abuse is a chronic disease and that treatment is a long-term process. The classic battle between clinician and client is to convince clients to acknowledge their addiction, seek adequate treatment, and pursue it sufficiently. Many of the lower-income addicts have few incentives (e.g., no job, home, or family to protect) and low personal motivation for seeking treatment. The facilities generally have Spartan accommodations, and some feature a good deal of confrontation. Clients often leave primary treatment prematurely and subsequently fail to utilize aftercare or self-help services.

Drug treatment often takes longer than one would suppose because recovery requires a period of gradual extinction of drug-related stimulus-response connections, personality adjustments, and a dramatic change in lifestyle if it is to be sustained. Drug abuser treatments have therefore included elements that go beyond the narrow limits of physiological withdrawal to include issues that are largely a function of the socioeconomic situation and psychological functioning of the client. Residential programs are often inexpensive replacements for jails, and clients go there as much for isolation from high-drug-rate neighborhoods and resocialization as for drug addiction treatment per se. Relapse rates for short-term detoxification programs are high, and relapse is an ever-present danger even after long periods of highly supportive treatment (e.g., as high as 50 percent following voluntary discharge from methadone maintenance). Treatment providers therefore stress the need for reimbursement of aftercare and long-term counseling. If length-of-stay targets are narrowly drawn as they are in other areas of medical care, they will ignore these clinical issues and will appear to providers to undermine recovery.

Quality of care.   The major obstacles to sustaining high levels of care in public facilities are community resistance and low levels of funding. Physical facilities are often run down. Staff turnover is high, and staff educational backgrounds and training are limited due to low salary levels. Many trained counselors have left for higher-paying jobs in the private treatment sector or in employee assistance programs. Many also leave the field when they find that salary levels are inadequate for a more mature professional.

Another obstacle to establishing standards of care has been the lack of adequate research on the efficacy and cost-effectiveness of the major modalities of treatment and the components of these complex treatment regimens. Even when compared to mental health and alcoholism treatment, the drug treatment field has had few randomized trials (Goldstein et al. 1984). Until recently, attempts at randomized clinical trials of drug abuse modalities were unsuccessful because of ethical concerns or recruitment problems, client dropout or follow-up difficulties (Bale et al. 1980). Clinical trials on short-term detoxification services have met with some success (Wilson et al. 1975), and randomized studies of drug abuse prevention and inpatient administration of medications are not uncommon. By contrast, there have been relatively few successfully completed randomized studies of long-term outpatient psychosocial treatments (Ashery and McAuliffe 1990), methadone maintenance (Newman and Whitehill 1979), or treatments offered primarily by residential or outpatient self-help organizations. In the absence of rigorous information on what constitutes effective treatment or what providers should do, it is hard to monitor staff performance or judge the adequacy of the designs of specific programs.

Since the establishment of the National Institute on Drug Abuse less than sixteen years ago, the federal government has funded increasing numbers of randomized clinical trials of drug abuse treatments, and the results of these studies should play an increasingly important role in deciding what elements of care should become standard. Once experimental evidence of effectiveness is available, the field should have less difficulty designing optimal treatment programs and convincing the public and regulators that the costs of care are worthwhile. However, the recent state support of acupuncture detoxification treatment in Massachusetts, when to our knowledge there are no randomized trials of its use in drug treatment, indicates that society is still unwilling to await definitive evidence before funding a new treatment. Unfortunately, once a treatment modality is widely funded, it becomes difficult to conduct randomized trials to evaluate its efficacy, and discontinuation is unlikely even if the research produces negative results.

Policy issues in the private sector

The greatest changes in the drug field have occurred in the private sector. Those changes stem from the spread of drug use among the middle class, the expansion of third-party coverage of substance abuse services, cost inflation, and the introduction of regulatory mechanisms designed to control costs. These issues are new to the drug field and are already causing disruptions similar to those that other segments of health care witnessed some time ago.

Middle-class drug use.   While the heroin epidemic of the 1960s and 1970s was spreading through the lower classes, there was a parallel epidemic involving the nonmedical use of so-called "soft" drugs, initially used by elite college students and then by the rest of society. Advocates of liberalizing attitudes towards drug use argued effectively that there was no hard evidence that experimental use of marijuana was harmful or that it could lead to addiction or use of addictive substances such as heroin or cocaine. The government's response was to set up a drug abuse prevention system targeted at marijuana use by suburban youth rather than to set up an adolescent drug treatment system that might treat addicts and prevent use of more dangerous drugs. Despite the assurances to the contrary, hundreds of surveys have since shown that most college and high school students moved beyond marijuana to experiment with one or more of the whole spectrum of drugs of abuse (Smart and Whitehead 1972; McAuliffe, Breer, White, et al. 1988).

Moreover, epidemiologists have also found that the more drug *use* there is, the more *abuse* (or addiction) there is (Smart et al. 1971). Studies have found a consistent distribution (approximately log-normal) of users across a continuum of severity. Of those who ever use drugs, most just try them once or twice, many use them occasionally, some use them regularly, and a few become abusers or addicts. The more people there are who use drugs once or twice, the more people there are who end up abusing. Consequently, since the number of users has grown dramatically across the entire spectrum, it is not surprising that we have also witnessed a dramatic increase in the number of abusers who need treatment.

Since the mid-1960s our high schools and colleges have graduated cohort after cohort of students with a large percentage of persons (from 33 to 80 percent) who have histories of illicit drug use (McAuliffe, Wechsler, et al. 1984) and a smaller percentage (about 5 percent) who have had drug problems. At the same time, society's oldest cohorts of nonusing workers were retiring and dying. Although drug use tends to decline as people age and become involved in their families and careers (Winick 1962, 1964; Waldorf 1973), a significant proportion of those who ever use nonmedical drugs continue to use or abuse them (McAuliffe, Breer, White, et al. 1988).

To see how extensive drug use has become after twenty years of this process, let us review some recent data. In 1987, we surveyed 5,000 randomly selected households in Rhode Island and found that a quarter of the general public (26 percent of persons age 12 and over, including some as old as 99) had tried a controlled drug nonmedically at least once in their lives, and that 10 percent had done so in the last year (McAuliffe, Breer, White, et al. 1988). Seventeen percent of the current users met clinical criteria for drug abuse.

Nonmedical drug use has permeated all social strata. Data from the Rhode Island study show that drug use is clearly age-graded, but that the age of users has increased steadily. There are no longer any differences in overall drug use rates in different ethnic groups, although the groups do have preferences for specific drugs. Males have long used illicit drugs more than females (McAuliffe 1975), but the gender gap has narrowed. College-educated, middle-class persons reported slightly higher incidence of cocaine use than did less educated groups (McAuliffe, Breer, White, et al. 1988), while the latter groups still reported the highest incidence of heroin addiction. A 1984 national study of employed young men showed that current drug use is found in every major occupation and industry group (Mensch and Kandel 1988).

Drug use has also invaded parts of society that are charged with control of the drug problem. A Supreme Court nominee admitted to having used marijuana. A recent article (Neuffer 1988) claimed that drug use by the police was undermining the war on drugs. Three years ago a survey of a random sample of 600 doctors and pharmacists in Massachusetts showed that 35 percent had used a drug nonmedically at some time in their lives and that 10 percent had done so in the last year (McAuliffe, Rohman, et al. 1986). When this use was added to traditional self-medication, a full 59 percent reported some nonprescribed use ever, and one-third said they had used in the past year. Our survey of student professionals in 1979 showed that student doctors used no more or less than other student professionals, with social work, counseling, and law students reporting the highest rates of nonmedical drug use (McAuliffe, Wechsler, et al. 1984). When we surveyed medical and pharmacy students again five years later, we found that the drug use rates had changed little except for a doubling of the rate of cocaine use from 20 percent to 39 percent (McAuliffe, Rohman, et al. 1986). It is clear that illegal drug use has steadily become a much larger and more pervasive problem than it was before the 1960s.

Fortunately, the most recent evidence indicates that this epidemic of use has peaked, and we have begun to witness declines in its consequences. Since 1980, yearly surveys of high school and college students have shown gradual declines in the amount of marijuana use (Rogers 1990; *NIDA Notes* 1989a). Cocaine use also began declining in 1987, and the 1988 NIDA household survey indicated a reduction of drug use (50 percent decline in current cocaine use) among youths (*NIDA Notes* 1989b). Because the consequences of drug use often do not respond until several years after changes in drug use prevalence (Hunt 1974), we have not yet seen declines in all of its consequences. For example, NIDA's Drug Abuse Warning Network (DAWN) found that cocaine-related emergency room admissions declined 30 percent during four consecutive quarters beginning in the third quarter of 1989, after admissions had increased in 15 of 16 previous quarters (Sobel 1990). Deaths due to cocaine use have continued to increase each year between 1985 and 1989, but the size of the increases have declined steadily (*NIDA Notes* 1990). Also, in the same year that Boston recorded a record level of homicides (Associated Press 1990), the number of cocaine samples seized and the volume of those samples declined for the first time in four years (Kennedy 1991).

Growth of the private drug treatment industry.   Because serious drug abuse is now a fact of life in the working and middle classes of this country, the private drug treatment field has undergone important changes. Employer and employee organizations have responded to the growing drug problem among their members. Employee assistance programs, which originally responded to the problem of alcoholism, have expanded their scope to include abuse of controlled drugs. Schools have adopted student assistance programs, which include case finding, counseling, referral for treatment, and follow-up as well as prevention. Unions have often been strong supporters of drug abuse programming. The American Medical Association and state medical societies have responded to physicians' drug and alcohol abuse problems by launching the impaired professionals movement, which now includes a wide range of professions in virtually every state.

Drug testing is growing rapidly in the workplace. Recent surveys indicate that 34 percent of Fortune 1000 companies are testing employees or job applicants, up from 25 percent just three years before (*Journal* 1988), although only 3 percent of employers in general have drug testing programs. The military has conducted drug testing for some time now and has reported great success in reducing the amount of drug use among the troops (Maltby 1988). Increasingly, other government agencies, such as the Department of Transportation and the National Aeronautics and Space Administration, have instituted drug screening programs, especially for workers in sensitive jobs (*EAP Digest* 1989). Recently the courts have begun to rule on the constitutionality of these procedures. It appears likely that testing will play an increasingly important role in the fight against drug abuse.

Despite the insurance industry's understandable reluctance to increase health benefits, private third-party payers now reimburse for substance abuse treatment in at least 37 states (McAuliffe, Breer, White, et al. 1988). In many instances this coverage had to be mandated by the states or pushed by employers with testing programs and union contracts that require counseling and treatment referrals. To compete, HMOs have added drug treatment to their benefit packages. This trend is growing steadily, although rising health care costs have recently resulted in eight states adopting low-cost plans that in some instances drop substance abuse benefits to make health insurance more affordable for lower-income populations (Freudenheim 1990).

Medicaid reimbursement is also being used more extensively for substance abuse treatment. For example, Massachusetts treatment programs, including methadone maintenance, detoxification, and residential rehabilitation facilities, can now draw upon Medicaid, which enjoys broad political support, rather than on drug treatment allocations, which have only limited political support.

As a result of the infusion of large amounts of new dollars, an industry of for-profit drug treatment facilities has developed. Where there were once just isolated sanitaria, there are now large national chains and many independent local facilities that advertise heavily and lobby to protect their interests. Excess hospital capacity is also being converted to drug detoxification facilities with strong medical emphases. Hospital beds for chemical dependency treatment more than doubled from 16,005 in 1978 to 34,364 in 1987 (*Addiction Report* 1989). Addictionology has become a medical subspecialty, no doubt in part a function of reimbursement trends and the presence of recovering physicians who want to help others.

Recognition that even heroin addicts are now capable of paying for treatment has led some states to develop for-profit methadone maintenance clinics. Critics in the field refer to these programs as "dosing for dollars" stations, because they often offer fewer counseling services than state-supported methadone programs.

In addition to the expansion of professional treatment services, there has been a phenomenal growth of the middle class—oriented self-help movement into the drug field. Ten years ago Boston did not have a single Narcotics Anonymous meeting. Today, like most major cities throughout the country, it has numerous meetings each night. There is a large recovery community that supports substance-free dances, drug-free housing, conferences of recovering people, vacation excursions for recovering people, and the like. The theories incorporated in these self-help programs have had a tremendous impact on the content of professional treatment as well. As is the case in the alcohol field, many drug counselors are themselves recovering persons who strongly support the twelve-step approach of Narcotics Anonymous (based on the Alcoholics Anonymous model). It is now more socially acceptable to be a recovering person, and the public is more inclined to feel that substance abuse is a disease for which treatment should be provided. The Betty Ford Center has become famous, and daily we learn of public disclosures of substance abuse by prominent people, such as the wife of former Massachusetts governor Michael Dukakis and Washington mayor Marion Barry.

All of the phenomena we have described are new to drug abuse over the past decade or so. As a result of these many changes in a heretofore sleepy field, policy development has been unable to keep up. Most of the reactions are only now taking form.

Policy and regulatory responses.   In contrast to the chronic shortage of funds that plagues drug treatment for the poor, the major health policy problem in the private sector is cost containment. In many states, insurers initially developed substance abuse benefit packages that were based on the medical model of drug abuse and that also attempted to control costs by reimbursing only inpatient or residential care. Less expensive outpatient care was either not covered at all or reimbursed minimally, and coverage was often insufficient to maintain gains achieved by clients during residential treatment. The result was that middle-class addicts, who were not physiologically dependent and who had home environments that made outpatient treatment feasible, entered expensive residential treatment centers.

States have recently moved to correct this problem. Certificate-of-need programs are being used in Rhode Island to control the growth of private residential treatment facilities. This process is exposing the field's limited technical ability to determine need, offer alternative outpatient forms and levels of care, and assess the cost-effectiveness of treatment and varying lengths of stay. In some cases regulatory mechanisms seem to be discouraging low-cost outpatient programs rather than higher-cost inpatient programs. Since residential facilities promise greater financial returns, investors in such facilities can more easily justify going through the expensive regulatory process. Massachusetts has consequently confined its determination of need program to inpatient treatment. There is, however, need for rational planning of the current expansion in order to use resources most efficiently and to avoid some of the inflationary pressures seen in other parts of the health care system.

Several technical developments over the past two decades promise to help solve some of these planning and regulatory problems. Epidemiological methods, including new measurement tools and cost-efficient survey techniques, have improved significantly, so that it is now possible to obtain more reliable estimates of the size and nature of the problem (McAuliffe, Breer, White, et al. 1988). More precise prevalence estimates should make it easier to apply rational drug abuse treatment planning models.

Advances in research methods for evaluating treatment services will also have an effect on policy development in the next decade. Whereas the major modalities of drug treatment (e.g., methadone maintenance) were implemented without first conducting randomized trials to establish their efficacy, recent studies have demonstrated that such trials are now technically feasible. A number of randomized trials in the alcohol field have direct relevance to the treatment of drug abuse (Annis 1985–86; Miller and Hester 1986), and similar studies for drug abuse treatment are forthcoming.

Levels of care.   It should come as no surprise that levels of care have become a major cost-containment issue for the field. In earlier times, heroin and alcohol addiction (both of which cause significant physiological symptoms) and clients' poor home environments together argued for inpatient (hospital or hospital-like) detoxification treatment, where one could receive medical monitoring followed by a period of residential "rehabilitation" treatment in a setting far from home. Today, however, many middle-class patients are addicted to cocaine, which does not require medical monitoring, and there are acceptable home situations for outpatient recovery. Unfortunately, many cost-cutting forms of intermediate care (halfway houses and evening care or day care) that would provide suitable substitutions for residential rehabilitation have not been reimbursable by third-party providers. Moreover, it has become apparent to many experts in the field that the traditional chemical dependency model was deficient in the amount of support it provided to recovering persons who were newly discharged from residential to ambulatory treatment. Studies show that most relapses occur soon after discharge to outpatient status. Drug abuse treatment, as distinct from alcoholism treatment, lacked a system of care (e.g., halfway houses or day care) offering a gradual reduction in the level of support. Pressures to reduce costs have already caused third-party payers (e.g., in Maryland) to reconsider their stance on reimbursement of intermediate forms of treatment.

In support of this challenge to the traditional chemical dependency treatment model, randomized clinical trials over several decades and different countries have found that outpatient alcohol treatment is as effective in the long term as inpatient alcohol treatment (Annis 1985–86; Miller and Hester 1986). Other studies have shown that many substance abusers, including heroin and cocaine addicts (Biernacki 1986; Schaffer and Jones 1989), can achieve recovery without any professional treatment whatsoever. Analysis of these cases shows that substance abusers employ the same methods of recovery as those recommended by professionals. By extension, these results suggest that outpatient and self-help drug treatment modalities could replace inpatient and residential treatment entirely in many instances. Debate is shaping up regarding the necessity of routine referral of substance abusers to residential treatment. The question has also spawned government-funded research programs on the "matching hypothesis," the claim that the negative results of randomized trials can be explained by the failure to match clients with appropriate treatment. Presumably, there are certain patients who need inpatient treatment, while others do not.

In the past, when residential treatment had to be paid for out of pocket, admission certification was a minor issue, since few substance abusers were directed to or sought treatment if they did not need it. Most did not obtain treatment even when they needed it. With third-party reimbursement now widely available, and with substance abuse treatment in inpatient settings becoming more accepted and perhaps even fashionable in some circles, more careful review of treatment necessity is needed. Certainly, the question of whether a client needs inpatient or outpatient care will be examined with increasing scrutiny. An implication of the new conditioning model of addiction is that we should learn to recognize the early stages of addiction and to get clients into treatment before they enter the end-stage of the disease, marked by advanced withdrawal symptoms. This feature should raise concerns for third-party payers that are dominated by medically oriented thinking and have a stake in keeping the eligible population within bounds.

Length of stay.   Issues concerning length of stay have only just begun to be addressed in this field, but they promise to produce substantial controversy. A sharp debate between industry interests, patient advocates, and federal officials developed several years ago when length-of-stay targets for inpatient alcohol detoxification were announced by federal authorities. Because the targets were substantially shorter than traditional lengths of stay, the federal standards were withdrawn while data were collected to support a defensible target. That battle is likely to be a model for similar discussions of length of stay for drug abuse services.

The same issues can be found in all the other major treatment modalities in the field. Inpatient rehabilitation treatment, which lasts 28 days by tradition, is expensive ($10,000 per episode is common), and many drug abusers require several treatment episodes before they can sustain recovery. The length of stay of residential treatment is already a target for cost containment, but the battle to control costs will not be an easy one, since this part of the industry has the greatest financial and political clout. For example, randomized trials of the length of inpatient services for alcoholism (which are often provided in the same facilities as drug treatment) have indicated that shorter stays would be more cost effective, but as yet this research is only beginning to have an impact on the field.

A major new development in the field is the concept of managed care. Third-party payers are using chemical dependency professionals in managed care companies to certify and monitor admissions, levels of care, and the length of stay of substance abuse patients in chemical dependency programs (Horwitz 1988). By the end of 1990, managed care was apparently having a major impact on the field and was on the front pages of industry publications (Meacham 1990).

Quality of care.   Unlike the public sector, where quality suffers due to lack of funds, the threats to quality in the private sector stem from the easy availability of funds, new treatment forms, and efforts at cost containment. With many new providers entering the field to take advantage of third-party reimbursement, one can anticipate that quality issues will soon attract increasing attention. It should also not be surprising that personnel certification has become a major movement, especially as large numbers of middle-class recovering persons enter the field without any formal training. Many long-time drug treatment experts have raised concerns about the capacity of alcoholism counselors in residential facilities to treat clients who abuse controlled drugs. Licensing of these facilities to provide both drug and alcohol treatment without further training of staff is also a policy concern.

New treatment forms lead to quality of care problems, since regulators are unclear what the essential elements of treatment are and what indicators need to be examined when they evaluate care. For example, state drug abuse administrations are not yet experienced in regulating for-profit methadone programs, and they must depend on each others' trial and error approaches to policing these new treatment forms.

Quality assurance systems, especially in community-based programs, are poorly developed in this field. In the past, quality assurance was largely confined to reviewing the adequacy of physical facilities and administrative records. Hospital-based programs are within institutions that have long experience with quality assurance issues and the resources to implement them in every department. Community-based programs are often small and lack the necessary expertise to conduct quality assurance. Little attention has been devoted to developing organizational mechanisms and methods of reviewing the content of treatment programs, the performance of counseling staff, or program revision in light of new developments in the field. For example, our own review of community drug-prevention programming in one state suggested that little had changed in the services provided, even though the research community had established somewhat convincingly that some of these approaches were not measurably effective. In our Rhode Island study we recommended the formation of a statewide treatment standards panel made up of clinicians, academics, third-party representatives, and state officials. One recommended goal of the panel was to organize reviews of community programs. The first meeting of the panel was held in early 1991.

The problems of quality will no doubt emerge as cost-containment measures, such as managed care, begin to have their effects. Patient advocates and providers have begun to complain that cost considerations are resulting in patients being denied admission to appropriate levels of care, especially residential treatment, or being discharged too soon (Meacham 1990). An early clash over cost containment and quality of care has involved substance abuse services provided by HMOs (*Managed Care Report* 1989: 6). Employee assistance programs were unhappy about attempts to limit the use of inpatient treatment and about the short lengths of outpatient counseling benefits offered by HMOs to their subscribers. Many employee assistance program counselors have themselves recovered by going through the traditional treatment system, and many have strong self-help traditions, which assume that recovery is a lifelong process, not something that can be treated adequately in a fixed number of counseling sessions. Providers in the substance abuse field will no doubt have just as much difficulty as providers in the rest of health care in accepting the notion that some increase in relapse rate is an inevitable consequence of efforts to eliminate inappropriate admissions or unnecessary lengths of stay. Obviously, there are major philosophical and practical differences to be resolved between these treatment providers and cost-conscious health care regulators.

Conclusions

The drug field has undergone enormous changes in the last several decades. Policy development has not kept up. Dramatic shifts in the size and nature of the problem since the mid-1960s have set the stage for many classic policy debates. The Nixon administration responded to an epidemic of heroin addiction in the early 1970s by establishing a system of state drug treatment systems, with methadone maintenance as a key modality of treatment. The heroin problem then appeared to stabilize, and there was even a brief period of excess treatment capacity in the public sector. Funding of services declined in inflation-adjusted dollars over the remainder of the 1970s, and the Reagan administration made significant cutbacks in funding while converting from direct funding of services to a state block grant mechanism in the early 1980s. Long waiting lists at publicly funded programs have been the norm in the 1980s. The crack epidemic has caused a rash of drug-related crime and an increase in demand for publicly funded drug treatment for the urban poor. The AIDS epidemic among intravenous drug users has put additional pressure on the public treatment system. As a result, the federal government has recently begun to make more resources available. Waiting lists persist at public treatment programs, however, in part because of state fiscal woes and local resistance to siting public drug facilities. Especially affected are methadone maintenance and AIDS-related programs.

Calls for legalization in response to the violent crimes produced by the crack epidemic appear to be acts of desperation rather than carefully developed policy proposals. With drug use declining steadily, it is quite likely that violent crime will also decline without our resorting to poorly thought-out, high-risk measures.

At the same time, drug use by middle- and working-class youth that began in the mid-1960s and climaxed with the epidemic of cocaine use has resulted in a large increase in the demand for drug treatment services and third-party reimbursement of these services. The model of treatment has been the 28-day residential treatment program exemplified by the Betty Ford Center. As more and more insurers have extended coverage to substance abuse services, often mandated by state legislatures, a new, nationwide private treatment industry has developed. Since treatment episodes cost $10,000 or more and several episodes are usually needed to sustain long-term recovery, the cost of drug treatment has grown rapidly. Debates over cost control and quality of care that are familiar elsewhere are just now emerging in the drug field, primarily with respect to managed care. The AIDS epidemic has added another ominous dimension to the debate. The next five years promise to be an interesting and tumultuous period in the drug treatment field.

References

Addiction Report. 1989. Beds for Treating Addiction Doubled. December, pp. 2–3.
Anglin, M. D., G. R. Speckart, M. W. Booth, and T. M. Ryan. 1989. Consequences and Costs of Shutting Off Methadone. *Addiction Behaviors* 14 (3): 307–26.
Annis, Helen. 1985–86. Is Inpatient Rehabilitation of the Alcoholic Cost Effective? Con Position. *Advances in Alcohol and Substance Abuse* 5 (1/2): 175–90.
Ashery, Rebecca, and William E. McAuliffe. Implementation issues and techniques in randomized trials of outpatient psychosocial treatments for drug abusers: Recruitment of subjects. Unpublished paper. Department of Psychiatry, Harvard Medical School at Cambridge Hospital, 1493 Cambridge Street, Cambridge, MA 02139.

Associated Press. 1990. Many Cities Setting Records for Homicides in Year. *New York Times*, 9 December, p. 141.

Bale, Richard N., W. Van Stone, J. Kuldau, T. Engelsing, R. Elashoff, and V. Zarcone. 1980. Therapeutic Communities Versus Methadone Maintenance. *Archives of General Psychiatry* 37: 179–93.

Biernacki, Patrick. 1986. *Pathways from Heroin Addiction: Recovery Without Treatment*. Philadelphia: Temple University Press.

Blumberg, Herbert H. 1976. British Users of Opiate-type Drugs: A Follow-up Study. *British Journal of Addictions* 71 (1): 65–67.

Budd, R. D., J. J. Muto, and J. K. Wong. 1989. Drugs of Abuse Found in Fatally Injured Drivers in Los Angeles County. *Drug and Alcohol Dependence* 23 (2): 153–58.

Campbell, Norman A., Charles Hachadorian, Jr., and Diane A. Tellier. 1990. *Results of Compliance with a State-Mandated Drug Incident Reporting System, Calendar Year 1989*. Providence: State of Rhode Island Department of Health.

Casadonte, Paul P., Don C. DesJarlais, Samuel R. Friedman, and John P. Rotrosen. 1990. Psychological and Behavioral Impact among Intravenous Drug Users of Learning HIV Test Results. *International Journal of the Addictions* 25 (4): 409–26.

Chu, A., L. S. Brown, S. Banks, T. Nemoto, and B. J. Primm. 1990. Intravenous Heroin Use: Its Association with HIV Infection in Patients in Methadone Treatment. In *Problems of Drug Dependence, 1989,* ed. L. Harris. Rockville, MD: National Institute on Drug Abuse.

Cook, D. R. 1987. Self-identified Addictions and Emotional Disturbance in a Sample of College Students. *Psychology of Addictive Behaviors* 1: 55–61.

Drug Abuse Warning Network. 1989. Table 2.06a: Drugs Mentioned Most Frequently by Emergency Rooms in 1988. In *Annual Data 1988: Data from the Drug Abuse Warning Network*. Rockville, MD: National Institute on Drug Abuse.

Dupont, Robert L., and Mark H. Greene. 1973. The Dynamics of a Heroin Epidemic. *Science* 181 (4101): 716–22.

EAP Digest. 1989. NASA to Use Drug Tests (*Detroit News*). March/April, p. 15.

Focus: A Guide to AIDS Research and Counseling. 1989. Heterosexual HIV Transmission. 4 (7): 1–4.

Freudenheim, Milt. 1990. States Try to Cut Cost of Insurance for Medical Care: Policies May Cover Less: Industry Says Cheaper Plans Are Geared for 33 Million Who Lack Protection. *New York Times*, 9 December, pp. 1, 34.

Gerstein, Dean R., and Henrick J. Harwood, eds. 1990. *Treating Drug Problems*. Vol. 1. Washington, DC: National Academy Press.

Glatt, Max M., David J. Pittman, Duff F. Gillespie, and Donald R. Hill. 1967. *The Drug Scene in Great Britain*. London: Arnold.

Goldstein, Michael S., Monica Surber, and Daniel M. Wilner. 1984. Outcome Evaluations in Substance Abuse: A Comparison of Alcoholism, Drug Abuse, and Other Mental Health Interventions. *International Journal of the Addictions* 19 (5): 479–502.

Graham, Renee. 1989. Lawrence Mayor's Tactics on Drugs Stir Rights Fears. *Boston Globe*, 27 June, pp. 13, 17.

Hachadorian, Charles, Jr., Norman A. Campbell, and Diane A. Tellier. Undated. *An Annualized Analysis of Drug-Related Incidents in Rhode Island Emergency Rooms, Calendar Year 1987.* Providence: State of Rhode Island Department of Health.

————. Undated. *An Annualized Analysis of Drug-Related Incidents in Rhode Island Emergency Rooms, Calendar Year 1988.* Providence: State of Rhode Island Department of Health.

Hadaway, Patricia, Barry L. Beyerstein, and J. Valda M. Youdale. 1991. Canadian Drug Policies: Irrational, Futile, and Unjust. *Journal of Drug Issues* 21 (1): 183–97.

Hasin, Deborah S., Bridget F. Grant, Jean Endicott, and Thomas C. Harford. 1988. Cocaine and Heroin Dependence Compared in Poly-drug Abusers. *American Journal of Public Health* 78 (5): 567–69.

Hohler, Bob. 1990a. Roadway Drug Testing Stirs Controversy in N.H. *Boston Globe*, 25 February, pp. 62–64.

————. 1990b. Cautions Raised on Sentences without Parole. *Boston Globe*, 16 December, pp. 57, 60.

Horwitz, Larry. 1988. Financial Factors Influencing Substance Abuse Treatment. *Managed Care Interface*, December, pp. 14–16.

Hunt, Leon Gibson. 1974. *Recent Spread of Heroin Use in the United States: Unanswered Questions.* Washington, DC: Drug Abuse Council.

Jackson, Derrick Z. 1989. Prisons Sitting on a Drug Bomb: Today's Inmates are Substance Abusers. *Boston Globe*, 28 May, pp. 75, 78.

The Journal. 1988. Employee Testing Up. 17 (1): 2.

Journal of NIH Research. 1989. Bennett's Battle Plan for the War on Drugs. 1 (4): 27–29.

Kennedy, John H. 1991. Budget Cuts, Dealer Savvy Hurt Drug War. *Boston Globe*, 21 January, pp. 21, 26.

Leavitt, Paul. 1991. Nationline: Economy, Drugs Top Urban Concerns. *USA Today,* 15 January, p. 3a.

Lehigh, Scot. 1990. Dukakis Says Education, not Police Key to Drug Fight. *Boston Globe*, 17 February, p. 22.

Maltby, Karin. 1988. Military's Drug-test Plans Ready but on Hold. *The Journal,* 1 July, p. 3.

Managed Care Report. 1989. Well-managed Outpatient Care Seen Best for Substance Abuse. 27 November, p. 6.

McAuliffe, William E. 1975. Beyond Secondary Deviance: Negative Labelling and Its Effects on the Heroin Addict. In *The Labelling of Deviance: Evaluating a Perspective,* ed. Walter R. Grove. New York: Sage.

————. 1980. A Test of Schur's Theory of Societal Drug Problems. In *The Labelling of Deviance: Evaluating a Perspective* (2nd ed.), ed. Walter R. Grove. Beverly Hills, CA: Sage.

————. 1982. Psychosocial Aspects of Therapeutic Addiction: Final Report. Unpublished report. Department of Behavioral Sciences, Harvard School of Public Health, Boston, MA 02115.

————. 1986. *Assessment of the Need for Drug Treatment Services in Massachusetts: Final Report.* Boston, MA: Drug Rehabilitation, Division of Commonwealth of Massachusetts.

McAuliffe, William E., Jeff Albert, Georgia Cordill-London, and Thomas K. McGarraghy. 1990–91. Contributions to a Social Conditioning Model of Cocaine Addiction. *International Journal of the Addictions* 25 (9a, 10a): 1145, 1181.

McAuliffe, William E., Paul Breer, Nancy White Ahmadifar, and Cathie Spino. 1991. Assessment of Drug Abuser Treatment Needs in Rhode Island. *American Journal of Public Health.*

McAuliffe, William E., Paul Breer, and Susan Doering. 1990. An Evaluation of Using Ex-addict Outreach Workers to Educate Intravenous Drug Users about AIDS. *AIDS and Public Policy* 4 (4).

McAuliffe, William E., Paul Breer, Nancy White, Cathie Spino, Lauren Goldsmith, Susan Robel, and Linda Byam. 1988. *A Drug Abuse Treatment and Intervention Plan for Rhode Island, Division of Substance Abuse.* Providence: State of Rhode Island.

McAuliffe, William E., and Robert A. Gordon. 1974. A Test of Lindesmith's Theory of Addiction: The Frequency of Euphoria Among Long-Term Addicts. *American Journal of Sociology* 79 (4): 795–840.

McAuliffe, William E., Mary Rohman, et al. 1986. Psychoactive Drug Use among Practicing Physicians and Medical Students. *New England Journal of Medicine* 315 (13): 805–10.

McAuliffe, William E., Henry Wechsler, Mary Rohman, et al. 1984. Psychoactive Drug Use by Young and Future Physicians. *Journal of Health and Social Behavior* 25 (1): 34–54.

McConnell, Harvey. 1991. Tracking Trends in Drug Policy: Legalization Proponents Anticipate Shifts to Their View. *The Journal* 20 (1): 16.

McKeganey, Neil. 1990. Being Positive: Drug Injectors' Experiences of HIV Infection. *British Journal of Addiction* 85 (9): 1113–24.

Meacham, Andrew. 1990. Treatment and Managed Care: An Uneasy Mix. *U.S. Journal of Drug and Alcohol Dependence* 15 (12): 1, 16.

Mensch, Barbara A., and Denise B. Kandel. 1988. Do Job Conditions Influence the Use of Drugs? *Journal of Health and Social Behavior* 29: 169–84.

Miller, William R., and Reid K. Hester. 1986. Inpatient Alcoholism Treatment: Who Benefits? *American Psychologist* 41 (7): 794–805.

Moore, Mark. 1990. Actually, Prohibition Was a Success. *2- IIHS Status Reports* 25 (1).

Murphy, Sean. 1990. Boston Police to Relocate Drug Control Unit. *Boston Globe,* 17 February, p. 18.

Musto, David. 1989. The History of American Drug Control. *Update on Law-Related Education* (13 (2): 3–6, 47, 54–56.

Nadelmann, Ethan A. 1989. Drug Prohibition in the United States: Costs, Consequences, and Alternatives. *Science* 245: 939–47.

National Institute on Drug Abuse. 1990. *National Household Survey on Drug Abuse: Main Findings, 1988.* Rockville, MD: National Institute on Drug Abuse.

Neuffer, Elizabeth. 1988. Addiction, Crime among Police Undercut Drug War. *Boston Globe,* 28 November, pp. 21, 33.

Newman, Robert G., and Walden B. Whitehill. 1979. Double-Blind Comparison of Methadone and Placebo Maintenance Treatments of Narcotic Addicts in Hong Kong. *Lancet,* 8 September, pp. 485–88.

NIDA Notes. 1989a. High School Seniors' Drug Use Hits Record Low. 4(2): 34.

————. 1989b. Americans' Current Illicit Drug Use Drops 37 Percent: NIDA's 1988 National Household Survey Also Reveals Continued Heavy Cocaine Use Among Frequent Drug Users. 4 (2): 42–43.

————. 1988–89. NIDA Launches $20 Million Program to Develop Addiction Treatment Drugs. 4 (1): 1–2.

————. 1990. The Two Faces of DAWN. 5 (4): 23.

Nyhan, David. 1990. The Unwinnable Propaganda War. *Boston Globe,* 15 February, p. 15.

O'Donnell, John A. 1969. *Narcotic Addicts in Kentucky.* Washington, DC: Government Printing Office.

Parade Magazine. 1989. Who Drinks? 24 December, p. 15.

Petitti, Diana, and Charlotte Coleman. 1990. Cocaine and the Risk of Low Birth Weight. *American Journal of Public Health* 80 (1): 25–28.

Pittman, Lahary. 1991. Acupuncture Treatment for Chemical Dependency and AIDS. Paper presented to the NIDA National Conference on Drug Abuse Research and Practice, Washington, DC, 12–15 January.

Rhame, Frank S., and Dennis G. Maki. 1989. The Case for Wider Use of Testing for HIV Infection. *New England Journal of Medicine* 320 (19): 1248–54.

Robertson, J. R., C. A. Skidmore, and J. J. K. Roberts. 1988. HIV Infection in Intravenous Drug Users: A Follow-up Study Indicating Changes in Risk-Taking Behaviour. *British Journal of Addiction* 83 (4): 387–91.

Rogers, Susan. 1990. NIDA's High School Senior Survey Also Provides Data on College Students' Drug Use. *NIDA Notes* 5 (4): 16–18.

Schaffer, Howard, and Stephany Jones. *Quitting Cocaine.* Cambridge, MA: Lexington.

Schur, E. 1962. *Narcotic Addiction in Britain and America.* Bloomington: Indiana University Press.

Schuster, Charles R. 1990. NIDA's Response to the GAO Report. *NIDA Notes* 5 (4): 3–5, 22.

Skorneck, Carolyn. 1989. Number of Prescription Drug Cases Down a Third. *Boston Globe,* 7 December, p. A2.

Smart, R. G., and P. C. Whitehead. 1972. The Consumption Patterns of Illicit Drugs and Their Implications for Prevention of Abuse. *Bulletin on Narcotics* 24 (1): 39–47.

Smart, R. G., P. C. Whitehead, and L. Laforest. 1971. The Prevention of Drug Abuse by Young People: An Argument Based on the Distribution of Drug Use. *Bulletin on Narcotics* 23 (2): 11–15.

Sobel, Kelly H. 1990. Cocaine-Related Hospital Emergency Room Visits Drop 30 Percent. *NIDA Notes* 5 (4): 6–7.

St. Louis, M. E., K. J. Rauch, L. R. Peterson, J. E. Anderson, C. A. Schable, and T. J. Dondero. 1990. Seroprevalence Rates of Human Immunodeficiency Virus Infection at Sentinel Hospitals in the United States. *New England Journal of Medicine* 323: 213–18.

Sweedler, Barry M. 1991. Drug Use among Fatally Injured Drivers of Heavy Trucks. Paper presented to the NIDA National Conference on Drug Abuse Research and Practice, Washington, DC, 12–15 January.

Tamura, M. 1989. Japan: Stimulant Epidemics Past and Present. *Bulletin on Narcotics* 41 (1 & 2): 83–93.

Terry, Charles E., and Mildred Pellers. 1928. *The Opium Problem.* New York: Bureau of Social Hygiene. Reprinted 1970, Montclair, NJ: Patterson Smith.

Verdone, Juliana. 1989. AIDS and Addicts: Is Testing a Rush to Judgment? *Boston Phoenix,* 22 September, pp. 12, 32, 34.

Waldorf, Dan. 1973. *Careers in Dope.* Englewood Cliffs, NJ: Prentice-Hall.

Weddington, William W., and Barry S. Brown. 1988. Acceptance of HIV-Antibody Testing by Persons Seeking Outpatient Treatment for Cocaine Abuse. *Journal of Substance Abuse Treatment* 5 (3): 145–49.

Wilson, B. K., R. R. Elms, and C. P. Thomson. 1975. Outpatient vs. Hospital Methadone Detoxification: An Experimental Comparison. *International Journal of the Addictions* 10 (1): 13–21.

Winick, Charles. 1962. Maturing Out of Narcotic Addiction. *Bulletin on Narcotics* 14 (1): 1–7.

———. 1964. The Life Cycle of the Narcotic Addict and of Addiction. *Bulletin on Narcotics* 16 (1): 1–11.

Mental Health Policy for the 1990s: Tinkering in the Interstices

M. Gregg Bloche and Francine Cournos

Abstract. That public policy has abysmally failed the chronically mentally ill seems beyond genuine dispute. Successive reforms have foundered on the familiar shoals of overblown expectations and insufficient resources. In this paper, we review current policies affecting the chronic and disabled mentally ill, and we consider some approaches to reform. We begin by trying to identify and characterize the chronically mentally ill and their disabilities. Next, we consider the chaotic patchwork of federal and state programs that has come to replace the asylum. We then criticize several competing models of reform that we believe fail to make an empathic connection with the mentally ill. Finally, we urge a strategy of limited reform consistent with available empirical data about program effectiveness and sensitive to the likely economic, political, and legal constraints of the 1990s.

Introduction

This paper focuses on the challenges for public policy posed by the chronic and disabled mentally ill. That American health policy has failed this group abysmally seems beyond genuine dispute. Over the last two centuries, successive tides of reform have promised to ameliorate the personal tragedy and social disruption wrought by chronic mental illness, only to founder on the familiar shoals of overblown expectations and grossly inadequate resources. Each reformist surge has left a lasting residue of "pessimism, retrenchment, and neglect" (Morrissey and Goldman 1984). In this paper, we review the current state of public policy toward the chronic and disabled mentally ill, and we assess some strategies for reform.

We begin by attempting to identify and characterize the chronically mentally ill and their disabilities. This task is made difficult by the ambiguities that

The authors are grateful to Daniel Ernst and Heathcote Wales for their comments on a previous draft. They also thank Lawrence Brown, William Eskridge, Jr., and Michael Seidman for their guidance and Judith Beach for her research assistance.

plague definitions of this group and the inconsistencies between different sets of epidemiological data. We then consider the incomplete story of "deinstitutionalization" and the chaotic patchwork of federal and state programs that came to replace the asylum. Next, we briefly address several competing models of reform that we dismiss for their failure to make an empathic connection with the actualities of severe mental illness. Finally, we urge a pragmatic approach to reform that we believe is grounded in empirical evidence and sensitive to the likely political, economic, and legal constraints of the 1990s.

Identifying the chronic and disabled mentally ill

Disorders and disabilities.   Recent epidemiologic studies suggest that upwards of 15 percent of Americans meet diagnostic criteria for one or another mental disorder (Kiesler and Sibulkin 1987) as defined by the drafters of the American Psychiatric Association's diagnostic manual (1987). But these "disorders" are, for the most part, not persistently and severely disabling. The number of Americans grossly impaired by chronic mental illness is much lower: 2.4 million, or about 1 percent of the U.S. population, according to the National Institute of Mental Health (U.S. DHHS 1980). Of these, 1.7 million are believed to maintain a state of moderate to severe disability for at least one year. Vagueness about the meaning of disability afflicts these estimates,[1] but they are useful as ballpark indicators.

It has been estimated that about 900,000 Americans are chronically institutionalized because of mental disability—150,000 in private, state, Veterans Administration, and other government-run inpatient psychiatric facilities and 750,000 in nursing homes (Goldman, Gattozzi, and Taube 1981). Of those in nursing homes, 400,000 suffer from organic dementias[2] and 350,000 from other chronic mental disorders. Up to 1.5 million more live in community settings—with families, in group living situations, in single-room-occupancy hotels, or on the streets (Morrissey and Goldman 1986).

The most common psychiatric diagnoses carried by men and women in the approximately 1 percent of the U.S. population deemed grossly impaired by

---

1. Psychiatric epidemiologists have been more successful in developing statistically reliable definitions of clinical syndromes than they have been in developing measures of disability.

2. Persons with organic dementias (most of whom are over 65 years old and not psychotic) present clinical and social problems very different from those of chronic patients with major psychiatric illnesses (e.g., bipolar disorder and the schizophrenias). We include them in these numbers for historical, not clinical, reasons. During the last decade of the nineteenth century and the first few decades of the twentieth, reform-minded state legislatures took on full fiscal responsibility for the institutionalized insane, and localities eagerly reconceptualized senility as a form of insanity in order to shift the burden of care for the demented elderly to the states. A large movement of demented patients from local almshouses to state mental hospitals ensued (Grob 1983). By the end of World War II, 30 percent of the residents of state hospitals were 65 or older (Council of State Governments 1950).

chronic mental illness are schizophrenia, schizoaffective disorder, and bipolar disorder (U.S. DHHS 1980). These patients usually suffer from repeated episodes of psychosis and poor intercurrent functioning, including irregular employment, unemployment, difficulties in social relationships, and poor nutrition and personal hygiene. Contrary to a widely held impression, very few pose a substantial risk of violence to others. Neither the developmentally disabled nor substance abusers without other, major psychiatric diagnoses are included in these estimates. Some Americans with dementing illnesses (e.g., Alzheimer's disease) and other organic syndromes are included. Because separate government programs (and different clinical strategies) address the problems of substance abusers, the developmentally disabled, and those with dementia and other organic mental impairments, we will not consider these groups here.

Mental illness and homelessness.   The incidence of chronic and disabling mental illness within America's growing population of homeless people is a sharply controverted issue. The heterogeneity of the homeless and formidable methodologic obstacles have made empirical research difficult. Data on homeless families, single women, and men and women who live in the streets instead of shelters are very limited. Surveys of the prevalence of psychiatric disorders among various homeless populations have yielded estimates ranging from 15 to 90 percent. The incidence of chronic and disabling psychiatric illness (primarily schizophrenia and major affective disorders) within populations of homeless men living in shelters has varied between 25 and 50 percent (Keogel et al. 1988). In eight studies of homeless shelter and street populations conducted over the last dozen years, rates of previous psychiatric hospitalization ranged from 20 to 35 percent (Gelberg et al. 1988). The American Psychiatric Association estimates a 40 percent prevalence for major mental illness (schizophrenia and major affective disorders) among homeless persons nationwide (Arce and Vergare 1984).

Despite this uncertainty, it is plainly wrong to conclude, as some mental health professionals have (Wilkinson 1983), that the problem of homelessness is largely a consequence of inadequately treated psychiatric illness. If the above epidemiologic data are even roughly reflective of reality, most homeless men and women do *not* suffer from chronic and disabling mental illness. Their homelessness is better understood as a consequence of social developments beyond the scope of this paper, including a sharp drop in the availability of low-rent housing, reductions in social welfare programs, and the increasing social and economic estrangement of the underclass (Ropers 1988).

Political powerlessness.   An outstanding characteristic of the chronically mentally ill as a group is their political impotence. Their limited social skills and personal disorganization render them uniquely ineffective as political actors in the struggle for social resources (Scull 1985). For those patients who overcome clinical adversity to function effectively in society, the stigma of mental illness is a powerful disincentive to personal activism on behalf of less fortunate peers (Mechanic 1985). Through the formation of lobbying groups, families of the chronically mentally ill have had some impact, but they have been inhibited by their often-marginal socioeconomic status, fear of stigma, and preoccupation with the burden of coping with disordered members (Scull 1985). For the chronically mentally ill and their advocates, competition for public attention and for prominence on the national agenda has yielded repeated frustration (Marmor and Gill 1986).

Even in court, where mental patients won notable civil rights victories as individuals in the 1960s and 1970s, the mentally ill *as a class* have fared poorly. Despite a history of stigmatization and political powerlessness comparable to that of vilified racial minorities, the mentally disabled have apparently been denied status as a "suspect" or even "quasi-suspect" classification for the purpose of judicial review under the equal protection clause of the U.S. Constitution. In rejecting the claim of the mentally retarded to status as a "quasi-suspect" class entitled to "heightened scrutiny" of legislation affecting them, the U.S. Supreme Court declared its unwillingness to extend this protection to "the disabled, the mentally ill," and other "groups who have perhaps immutable disabilities," who fare poorly in politics, and who "can claim some degree of prejudice from at least part of the public at large."[3] Thus the mentally ill are ineligible for the heightened judicial protections against discriminatory state action guaranteed to racial minorities and to women.

The tragic incompleteness of "deinstitutionalization" policy

Thirty years ago, many, perhaps most, of the chronic and disabled mentally ill spent years of their lives in state and county mental hospitals. In 1955, according to the National Institute of Mental Health, the population of state and county asylums peaked at almost 560,000 (Kiesler and Sibulkin 1987). "Asylum" was once an ideal—advocates of "moral treatment" from the 1820s through the 1850s urged that the insane be protected from the stresses of society and be given individualized spiritual guidance and support (Rothman 1971). But by the late nineteenth century, this ideal had worn thin. State asylums had become grossly overcrowded and essentially custodial (Rothman 1980).[4]

---

3. City of Cleburne, Texas v. Cleburne Living Center, 473 U.S. 432, 445 (1985). It should be noted that in Cleburne, which involved a zoning ordinance requiring a special use permit for the operation of a group home for the mentally retarded, the Court invoked the once-moribund "rational basis" test to reject this requirement as an expression of "irrational prejudice" against the mentally retarded. Id. at 450.

4. From the 1820s through the 1850s, advocates of "moral treatment" pressed the states and

The story of "deinstitutionalization" over the last several decades is well known, and we will not retell it here, but we will highlight several elements that have received insufficient attention.

Transinstitutionalization. The term "deinstitutionalization" is seriously misleading. The presence of 750,000 mentally disabled persons in nursing homes at the start of the 1980s (Goldman, Gattozzi, and Taube 1981) suggests that there has been large-scale *transinstitutionalization*. More than half of all nursing home residents suffer from chronic mental illness, though most of these also have disabling medical problems (Kiesler and Sibulkin 1987).[5] After Congress amended the Social Security Act in 1960 (Medical Assistance to the Aged) and 1965 (Medicaid) to authorize state use of federal funds on a matching basis to pay for nursing home care, some states seized on the chance to shift custodial care costs to the federal government by transferring elderly asylum residents to nursing homes. Between 1955 and 1969, California reduced its population of elderly state hospital patients by 74 percent (Lerman 1985).

However, many states were much less responsive to this opportunity (ibid.). Based on an extensive review of the empirical literature on the clinical characteristics of nursing home residents, Kiesler and Sibulkin (1987) conclude that only a minority of the mentally ill in nursing homes today would have been state asylum residents before deinstitutionalization. Moreover, they note that the rate of increase in the chronically mentally ill population in nursing homes over the last few decades has been much greater than the rate of increase in the number of elderly persons in the general population. The migration of mentally ill persons to nursing homes during this period probably represents,

---

the federal government to construct public asylums for the insane poor. In 1854, both houses of Congress passed legislation to finance a large-scale federal asylum program, but President Franklin Pierce invoked his veto, insisting that the mentally ill were a state responsibility (Foley and Sharfstein 1983).

By the 1890s, state asylums had evolved into large, custodial institutions, beset by gross resource inadequacies and vast numbers of indigent residents. The ideal of moral treatment had been eclipsed by a professional ethos of therapeutic nihilism. In the first decade of the twentieth century, a new, medically oriented generation of reformers advocated a new kind of inpatient facility—the "psychopathic hospital"—to be affiliated with a university research and teaching program. State-supported psychopathic hospitals provided intensive treatment for a relative few, based on state-of-the-art ideas about psychotherapy and the biology of mental diseases, but this reform wave garnered insufficient fiscal and professional support to benefit the great mass of residents in custodial state facilities (Rothman 1980).

The third reform wave—the deinstitutionalization and community support movement of the 1960s and 1970s—foundered in the 1980s, for reasons discussed in this paper.

5. Studies of the incidence of psychiatric illness among nursing home patients have yielded variable results. An examination of Medicaid utilization review records for several thousand nursing home residents in Utah found that only one-third carried psychiatric diagnoses, though more than half of these had psychotic symptoms (Schmidt et al. 1977).

in part, the *neoinstitutionalization* of elderly and infirm persons once cared for in the community.[6]

Transinstitutionalization of another sort, involving younger patients, is reflected in a dramatic rise in the annual number of inpatient psychiatric days in general medical hospitals. Between 1969 and 1982, this number rose 116 percent, from 9.76 million to 21.12 million, reflecting an increased tendency to manage the chronically mentally ill with short-term, crisis-oriented hospitalizations in lieu of long-term state hospital residency (ibid.). Medicaid pays for many of these hospital stays, but many others are supported by local government subsidies to private hospitals for indigent care or by privately insured persons (indirectly) via cross-subsidies built into hospital rate structures.

Evidence from comparative clinical outcome studies[7] generally supports the conclusion that short-term hospitalization is less effective in the long run than are well-organized community treatment programs (Braun et al. 1981), although hospitalization is generally indicated when treatable psychiatric illness immediately endangers the patient's or another person's life. But clinical standards of care have been shaped in large measure by the resistance of private and public third-party payers to outpatient treatment for mental illness. The result, even for persons lacking inpatient insurance coverage, has been a strong professional bias in favor of hospital treatment. This preference is rendered especially resistant to contrary empirical evidence by clinical training that emphasizes emulation of senior practitioners' decision patterns (Friedman 1985).[8]

The reluctance of insurers, including Medicaid (Frank and Kessler 1984), to provide coverage for outpatient care is rational, given the broad discretion of clinicians and patients to determine "need" for treatment under most mental health insurance schemes. For inpatient care, the "moral hazard" problem of insurance is mitigated by powerful disincentives unrelated to hospital charges.

---

6. A comparative survey of nursing homes and mental hospitals found the two types of facilities indistinguishable with respect to central features of "total institutions" (Shadish and Bootzin 1984) as described by Goffman (1961).

7. Available hospitalization outcome data are problematic as a guide to policymaking because of lack of clarity about treatment methodologies and characteristics of patient populations in reported studies. Conflicting criteria for success further complicate the interpretation of outcome data. Optimal hospital treatment models for particular psychiatric conditions have yet to be defined (Cournos 1987b). Interpretation of outcome data for community treatment programs presents similar problems. Comparative outcome studies are thus unlikely to provide definitive policy guidance in the foreseeable future.

8. Friedman suggests another, powerful source of clinicians' inpatient bias: the inevitable feelings of hate and helplessness evoked by many severely ill patients. Some aggressive, sadistic, and suicidal patients elicit anger in practitioners, precipitating unconsciously punitive hospitalization decisions. Some depressed and seemingly helpless patients evoke feelings of hopelessness and helplessness in clinicians, leading to hospitalization as an expression of desperation.

These disincentives include stigma, deprivation of liberty, and such devastating possibilities as job loss and abandonment by stunned friends, family members, and other social supports. For outpatient treatment, stigma is much attenuated (and absent when confidentiality is maintained), and these other possibilities are generally negligible. The vagueness and subjectivity of psychiatric diagnosis ensure willing patients and their caretakers of only weakly constrained access to outpatient coverage. To the extent that indigent patients with incomplete outpatient coverage opt against outpatient care yielding benefits—e.g., improved quality of life and social functioning—that do not accrue to insurers by reducing their costs, the casualty insurance model generates a socially suboptimal level of outpatient treatment.[9]

Federal entitlement programs: Policy by coincidence.   The advent of antipsychotic drugs, a series of court decisions protecting patients' civil liberties, and heightened popular suspicion of large institutions are often mentioned as key factors in the depopulation of state asylums. But evidence suggests that the most immediate and powerful impetus was fiscal. Two-thirds of the national decrease in the state and county asylum population, from almost half a million people to less than 200,000, occurred between 1965 and 1975 (Kiesler and Sibulkin 1987),[10] the years of most rapid growth in federal entitlement programs for the disadvantaged. Medicaid, supplemental security income (SSI), social security disability insurance (SSDI), and other social welfare programs presented the states with an unprecedented opportunity to shift custodial care costs to the federal government (Mechanic 1987).

We have already mentioned the role of Medicaid in the relocation of elderly patients from state hospitals to nursing homes after 1965. In 1972, the inauguration of SSI, a federally guaranteed maintenance income stream for disabled persons, gave deinstitutionalization new impetus. The decisive role of entitlement streams, especially Medicaid and SSI, is suggested by the remarkable correlation between their availability and annual rates of state hospital population reduction. From 1960 to 1964, these rates averaged 2.1 percent, but between 1964 and 1972 they averaged 7.5 percent. For 1972–1974, the average was 10.8 percent (Lerman 1985). Though not specifically designed for the mentally ill, the new federal entitlement programs appear to have had a greater impact on their care than has any explicitly formulated state or federal mental health policy. The lack of attention to the impact of these programs

---

9. This assumes that indigent patients lack the financial or psychological capacity to value such benefits adequately in the marketplace through their purchasing behavior.

10. Between 1965 and 1975, according to NIMH data, the population of state and county mental hospitals decreased by 284,000, from 475,000 to 191,000. This drop represents 65 percent of the decline from 559,000 in 1955 (the peak year) to 125,000 in 1981 (Kiesler and Sibulkin 1987).

on the mentally ill had its consequences in the community. Many of the chronically mentally ill discharged from state hospitals entered living situations, such as single-room-occupancy "hotels" (SROs) and for-profit board-and-care homes, that offered minimal social support or supervision and poor access to clinical services (Goldman et al. 1981). By the late 1970s, monies provided to the mentally ill via Medicaid, SSI, and other entitlement streams totalled many times more than funds spent by states and the federal government to support mental health services.

Treatment in the community: The politics of neglect.   The failure of state mental health agencies, the federal government, and involved private institutions to buttress deinstitutionalization with adequate outpatient care and community support networks belies easy explanation. It is a mistake to attribute this failure, as some have, to supposed assurances from mental health professionals in the 1950s and early 1960s that the psychopharmacologic revolution would by itself solve the problems of the severely mentally ill. In fact, psychiatrists and other professionals with influence over policy were well aware by the late 1950s that the large-scale movement of treatment for chronic patients from the asylum to the community could not be effectively accomplished without the development of comprehensive aftercare and support programs (Gronfein 1985; Foley and Sharfstein 1983).

Nevertheless, state governments embraced the idea of deinstitutionalization as a way to reduce their mental health care expenditures, which included $1.2 billion annually for inpatient care by 1961 (Foley and Sharfstein 1983). The development of comprehensive outpatient treatment programs at taxpayer expense generated little interest among state legislators. No active constituency pressed state legislatures for new, large-scale outpatient treatment initiatives. For the reasons discussed earlier, patients and their families, then as now, lacked the capacity to focus the political process on their needs. With the exception of a few innovators (Milbank Memorial Fund 1962), state mental health agency leaders, who had built their careers in institutional psychiatry, displayed little enthusiasm for outpatient programs. Professional and lay community mental health activists, the constituency most committed to outpatient care, viewed state mental health authorities as the agents responsible for the evils of custodial inpatient care (Mechanic 1987). Having defined itself in opposition to the abuses bred by state-administered custodial care, the community mental health movement looked to the federal government for new outpatient initiatives.

By the early 1960s a broad coalition of reform-minded professionals and community activists had generated an unprecedented level of national political interest in mental health concerns. In 1961, a bipartisan mental health policy commission created by Congress several years earlier urged development of a national network of community mental health clinics, to be supported by a tripling of government spending for mental health services over the next ten years (Foley and Sharfstein 1983). Nurtured by the growing civil rights consciousness of the times (Mechanic 1987), devastating academic criticism of institutional psychiatry (Goffman 1961), and an emerging interest in the potential of community participation as a solution to myriad social ills (Starr 1982), the community mental health services model gained currency and was embraced by the Kennedy administration.

Advocates of the community mental health model proposed a diverse range of activities, including supportive care for the chronically mentally ill. But their primary focus was the prevention of mental disease and distress through community interventions designed to strengthen family and community relationships and to diminish citizens' sense of isolation and powerlessness (Rochefort 1984). As David Mechanic (1987) perspicaciously notes, this social conception of mental illness was mostly accepted on faith. Its idealistic adherents tended to overlook the severe psychosocial disabilities symptomatic of chronic mental illness and the implications of these disabilities for appropriate community treatment.

Proposals for the development of community services through federal aid to state mental health agencies foundered on the poor reputation of state hospitals and the consequent unpopularity of state agencies. In the politics that culminated in the 1963 passage of the Community Mental Health Centers (CMHC) Act, advocates of local community action triumphed over those who sought to place the locus of responsibility in state agencies. The 1963 act and its 1965 amendments made funds for construction, other start-up costs, and staffing directly available to not-for-profit community groups. Overall regulatory and administrative authority for the new program was vested in the National Institute of Mental Health (NIMH) (Foley and Sharfstein 1983).

The CMHC program had a diffuse range of goals, reflecting the alliance of interests that made possible its enactment. Aftercare for chronic patients competed with myriad other activities, including psychotherapies for those with less serious emotional problems and a variety of liaison and training programs for clergy, police, teachers, and even the courts. The activist community leaders and mental health professionals who oversaw and staffed individual centers displayed a greater interest in these latter, less traditional mental health activities (Rochefort 1984). Subsequent federal legislation renewing operating support for the CMHC program never mandated a greater commitment to the needs of the severely and chronically mentally ill.

The ideal of community self-determination that animated the CMHC program had a less than salutary impact on the development of CMHC services for the chronically mentally ill. NIMH policy endorsed the principle of local definition of problems as the best way to serve community needs and as empowering (and therefore health-promoting) in itself. But the political marginalization and powerlessness of the chronically mentally ill severely limited their influence in the process of community definition of problems and priorities. The CMHCs' autonomous governing boards, composed of local civic leaders and socially conscious professionals, tended to overlook the needs of the most severely ill (Greer and Greer 1984).[11]

State governments, sore losers in the struggle for federal mental health dollars, made this problem worse. State plans for the care of the chronically mentally ill outside the asylum failed to incorporate the nascent network of CMHCs. In some states, old legal barriers to the provision of clinical services by private, not-for-profit entities like CMHCs were maintained. A number of states refused to allow use of their funds to reimburse CMHCs for clinical services (ibid.). Sustained tension between the states and the CMHC program rendered federalism an instrument of inefficiency and waste.

Perhaps ironically, as Martha Burt and Karen Pittman (1985) contend, the Reagan administration's successful 1981 initiative to eliminate federal funding for community mental health centers and to substitute unrestricted "block grants" to state mental health agencies (equivalent to only 75 percent of the total previously awarded to the CMHC program) has had little adverse impact on care for the chronic and disabled mentally ill. In the 1980s, state mental health agencies have made outpatient services for the chronically mentally ill a higher priority than did the CMHCs in the 1960s and 1970s (Durman et al. 1984). This commitment contrasts notably with the institutional psychiatry bias that animated the state agencies a generation ago.

Leveraged by funds available from state agencies via the "block grants" program, this change in state priorities has forced changes in the CMHCs, which have become much more dependent on state contracts and grants.[12] A recent study, based on survey and interview data, of 76 CMHCs in 15 states found that state funding constituted half of the revenues of these facilities by 1984 (Larsen 1987).[13] While overall staffing levels declined and community consultation and education services were cut drastically between 1982 and 1984, many of these centers reassigned and added staff to programs serving the chronically mentally ill. Nearly all the centers reported that services for the chronically mentally ill had *expanded*. Increased staff time was devoted to comprehensive case management and to outpatient psychopharmacologic treatment and supportive psychotherapy for chronically disabled patients.

---

11. In this, the story of the CMHC movement and the chronically mentally ill is just another expression of the recurring tension in American social policy between the attraction of local community empowerment and the danger of community neglect of the most marginalized and needy.

12. CMHCs' other major income sources are fees paid by patients and reimbursement from Medicaid and private health insurance plans.

13. In contrast, direct federal support for these facilities dropped from 20 percent of annual revenues in 1982 to 2 percent in 1984 (Larsen 1987).

Community residential programs (halfway houses, group homes, shared apartments, lodges) added beds.

A related study of many of the same centers found that day treatment programs with an emphasis on psychosocial and vocational rehabilitation were expanding rapidly (Jerrell and Larsen 1984). CMHC managers acknowledged openly that state-funded and -administered reimbursement opportunities were a primary impetus for this growth. Increasingly, CMHCs are becoming integrated into statewide systems of care for chronic patients. Concludes one veteran student of CMHCs, "The . . . idea of a comprehensive, community-based mental health treatment agency is giving way to the emergence of a community-based institution for long-term clients" (Larsen 1987). Yet the availability of outpatient care for these clients still falls woefully short of clinical need.

Entitlement programs in the 1980s: Slashing the safety net.   Changes in the entitlement programs that once financed deinstitutionalization have had a less benign impact on the chronically mentally ill. The appearance of large numbers of mentally disabled homeless persons on our city streets in the 1980s coincided not with the emptying of state hospitals but with the decreasing real dollar value of entitlement streams (especially relative to housing costs) and the creation of formidable obstacles to eligibility. In the 1960s and 1970s, flexible administrative procedures and generous statutory construction eased access to SSI, SSDI, and other entitlements that assured mental patients of a minimal level of food and shelter outside the asylum (Foley and Sharfstein 1983). The Reagan administration's campaign to cut billions of dollars from SSI and SSDI in the early 1980s left this safety net badly damaged.

Changes in the administration of SSI were the most destructive.[14] By the late 1970s, about 375,000 chronically mentally ill persons—one-fourth of the estimated 1.7 million chronically mentally ill persons in the U.S.—were receiving SSI benefits (Burt and Pittman 1985). In March 1981, the Social Security Administration (SSA) began an aggressive program of SSI and SSDI eligibility redetermination, applying more stringent standards and procedures than had previously been employed. A year before, Congress had authorized triennial redeterminations, but the stricter standards and procedures were the SSA's invention. Nearly half of the cases reviewed led to determinations of ineligibility, and the mentally ill were disproportionately hard hit. Their difficulties with complicated paperwork and other, unforgiving procedural requirements made them particularly vulnerable (Goldman and Gattozzi 1988). The number of chronically mentally ill SSI and SSDI recipients denied benefits

---

14. The impact of cutbacks in SSI and SSDI was made even harsher by the disappearance of low-cost inner-city housing.

nationwide as a result of the SSA's redetermination program is unknown. But it has been estimated that in fiscal year 1982, 5,500 mentally ill beneficiaries were cut from the SSI roles in New York State, where about 10 percent of the nation's SSI and SSDI recipients live (Burt and Pittman 1985).[15] Extrapolating from these numbers to a nationwide estimate of 50,000 is a statistically dubious undertaking, but it provides a crude approximation.

Most of the adverse redeterminations were eventually reversed on appeal, but only after months without benefits. The consequences were frequently devastating—e.g., inability to pay rent, homelessness, and recurrence of psychotic symptoms. Stricter standards of disability were also applied to first-time determinations of eligibility, through policy manual changes not submitted to the administrative rulemaking process (ibid.). Eventually, adverse court action,[16] publicity about personal tragedies, and a firestorm of public criticism forced the SSA to back away from its harsh approach (Goldman and Gattozzi 1988). But eligibility for SSI (and SSDI) remains more difficult to achieve and to maintain than it was before 1981. Simultaneous cutbacks in state and local entitlement programs have hardly buffered this change.

Demographic change amplified the impact of these developments. Gentrification in the inner cities, accelerated by the coming of age of the "baby boom" generation, reduced the availability of SROs and other low-cost housing. Moreover, because schizophrenia, bipolar disorder, and schizoaffective disorder generally develop in early adulthood, the baby boom cohort added to the numbers of the psychiatrically disabled even as it swelled the ranks of their wealthier competitors in urban housing markets.

A failure of empathy

A chaotic patchwork of policy.   For the chronic and disabled mentally ill, the overall picture of policy today is a chaotic and incomplete patchwork of short-term inpatient units in government and private hospitals (oriented toward acute psychotic decompensations); inadequate outpatient psychiatric care provided by poorly coordinated clinics operated by states, local government bodies, and myriad for-profit and voluntary entities; and a fragmented assortment of entitlement programs, each with its own bureaucratic hurdles. In New Haven, Connecticut, for example, an indigent and mentally disabled person must negotiate up to thirteen different application procedures for federal, state, and

---

15. The proportion of this population that might qualify as chronically mentally ill is unclear from this report. Thus the significance of this estimate as an indicator of the impact of SSI redeterminations on the chronically mentally ill is uncertain.

16. Mental Health Ass'n of Minnesota v. Schweiker, 554 F. Supp. 157 (1982) (SSA disability standards that assumed capacity of mentally impaired persons age 18 to 49, without a *listed* impairment, to work found in violation of the Social Security Act and implementing regulations).

city health and welfare benefits.[17] Many of these programs have periodic review procedures with provisions for termination of benefits to those who do not complete the necessary paperwork.

This situation nurtures tragedy. Consider the plight of a schizophrenic male functioning marginally in the community who misses a filing deadline for review of his disability benefits, learns that his benefits have been terminated, and begins to decompensate psychiatrically. His next outpatient clinic appointment is still weeks away, and he is not enrolled in a comprehensive day treatment program. Thus the early signs of recurrent psychosis are not recognized by anyone with the capacity to direct him to emergency treatment. Over the next week, he becomes floridly delusional. Unable to negotiate the bureaucracy that has denied him his benefits, he loses his income and then his place in a single-room-occupancy hotel. Homeless and delusionally paranoid, he fails to show up at the clinic weeks later for his scheduled appointment. The clinic lacks the resources to respond by sending staff into the community to find and reengage him. The downward spiral ends, perhaps, when some minor street transgression catches the attention of a police officer who brings him to a hospital emergency room. For clinicians who work in urban psychiatric emergency departments, this is the stuff of daily life. Community residences, intensive outpatient clinical programs designed to detect and treat early signs of psychotic decompensation, and high-quality social and occupational rehabilitation programs are in notoriously short supply.

Policy as a tool for emotional disconnection.   In recent years, several appealing caricatures of the problem of chronic mental illness have informed policy and rationalized abdication. We consider them here because they have a way of recurring; for they are powerfully attractive as tools for disconnecting society from the disturbing incomprehensibility of madness and for avoiding the burden of helping those afflicted while recognizing their humanity.

One such caricature depicts mental illness as an exclusively biological problem, amenable only to biological interventions such as medication and electroconvulsive therapy. The policy implied by this portrayal is one of restraint bordering on abdication: state-of-the-art psychopharmacologic and other somatic treatment should be made readily available, but psychosocial and other rehabilitation programs are irrelevant to the problem and waste money better spent on biological research. This caricature is clinically blind and scientifically misleading. Schizophrenia and bipolar disorder are clearly disorders of the brain. Vulnerability to these disorders has a substantial genetic component

---

17. Interview with N. Heenani, April 1989. These benefits include SSI, SSDI, city welfare (a rent subsidy plus a small biweekly stipend), state welfare, state disability, Aid to Families with Dependent Children (AFDC), food stamps, and state subsidies for clothing, an apartment security deposit, fuel, a telephone, moving expenses, and transportation.

(Tsuang and Vandermey 1980), and current biological treatments can suppress some of the most dramatic symptoms, such as hallucinations and delusions. In some schizophrenic patients, brain tissue loss has been demonstrated (Weinberger et al. 1979), and other potential biological markers continue to generate research interest (Bowers 1980). But our developing understandings of the physiological substrate of psychiatric illness hardly imply the irrelevance of psychosocial understandings and interventions.

Schizophrenia, for example, is characterized by information-processing deficits (Braff and Saccuzzo 1985) and disturbances of arousal, attention, and higher-level executive functions of the mind (Anderson et al. 1986). Schizophrenics are impaired in their ability to cope with the expression of emotion in family relationships (Vaughn and Leff 1976). Psychotherapy, family education, occupational and social rehabilitation, and other psychosocial interventions sensitive to these deficits make a demonstrable difference by reducing recurrence of psychosis and improving patients' quality of life and social and occupational functioning (Cournos 1987a). Moreover, patient compliance with psychiatric medications depends vitally on the ability of clinic staff to engage patients in treatment. The continuing advance of neurobiology is unlikely ever to render psychological and social understandings of pathologic mental life irrelevant to human purposes. As some artificial intelligence workers have suggested, an understanding of the workings of an intelligent system at its lowest levels (e.g., machine language for computers or molecular interactions in biological systems) is not inherently relevant to understanding the system's highest levels—its processing of complex ideas and even emotions.

Another narrative means for insulating society from the suffering of the chronically mentally ill is portrayal of their problems as primarily the consequence of societal and professional hostility toward deviance (Szasz 1963). This narrative identifies as the central task of mental health policy the reining in of repressive responses to deviance. The possibility that forms of deviance conceptualized by society as severe mental illness might entail human misery even in the absence of an authoritarian social response is relegated to the periphery of political concern. This portrayal of the problem of mental illness appeals powerfully to the rights consciousness of American liberals, and the civil liberties issues it highlights merit continuing attention. The sensitivity of some mental health professionals to their patients' liberties remains insufficient (Ennis 1972). But to make civil liberties and the control of authority the *central* focus of mental health policy is to block empathic connection to the distress of the chronically mentally ill.

A third descriptive means for disconnection is statement of the problem as one of failure to take needed measures to coerce patients into treatment (Lamb and Mills 1986). This narrative portrays the homeless mentally ill as proof of the failure of deinstitutionalization. Flying in the face of empirical work supporting the conclusion that all but a small minority of the chronically mentally ill can be voluntarily engaged in treatment, this portrayal invites poli-cymakers to withdraw from the work of developing comprehensive community treatment and support programs capable of engaging patients. It overlooks the possibility that for some of the homeless mentally ill who chronically resist treatment, alienation may have followed unsuccessful efforts to find help. It invites a focus on the wording of civil commitment laws and on the admin-istrative details of coercion. The distracting power of the coercion focus has been illustrated dramatically in New York City, where former mayor Edward Koch's initiative to pick chronically mentally ill people off the streets against their will led to the Joyce Brown case, which for months monopolized public discussion in New York about the homeless mentally ill.

A fourth narrative of disconnection romanticizes the days when hundreds of thousands of the chronically mentally ill were housed in state custodial facilities (Schussheim 1989). It overlooks the dismal character of life in these institutions before depopulation began. It is insensitive to the unremitting problems of large-scale, custodial confinement of human beings—environ-ments that require mass behavior and foster personal regression, isolation from family and friends, and myriad staffing difficulties (Okin 1983). If the opin-ions of patients themselves were weighed, we would not consider a return to the care that existed then. In Segal and Aviram's (1978) moving account of deinstitutionalized patients functioning only marginally in the community, in board-and-care homes in California in the early 1970s, many admitted some degree of dissatisfaction, but 84 percent said they would object to returning to a mental hospital.

Clinical opportunities and political possibilities

Empirical evidence.   The opportunity exists for mental health policy to ad-vance beyond these inadequate descriptions toward an empathic reconnection with the chronically mentally ill. We can start by acknowledging what multiple empirical studies have shown over the last fifteen or so years. Community treatment and support programs that effectively coordinate living arrange-ments, psychiatric care, and social and vocational rehabilitation programs sen-sitive to the known deficits of persons with severe and chronic mental illness substantially improve social functioning and greatly enhance quality of life (Kiesler and Sibulkin 1987). Comprehensive case management, close mon-itoring of symptoms and medication side effects, psychotherapy strategies that emphasize educating patients about their illnesses, family counseling aimed at diminishing expressed emotion and overinvolvement (Anderson et al. 1986), and low-stress residential and "day hospital" programs built around the cognitive and emotional disabilities of the most common chronic illnesses (Cournos 1987a) can make possible the community management of the most severe psychiatric disorders. "Cure" is generally an unrealistic goal; gains from intensive community support and treatment programs tend to diminish with time after treatment is discontinued, suggesting the need to view such programs as a maintenance strategy for lifelong disability (Test and Stein 1978).

Comparative empirical studies have reached conflicting conclusions about whether such programs are cheaper to operate than the more typical practice—much less intensive outpatient (often only pharmacologic) care punctuated by crisis hospitalizations (Kiesler and Sibulkin 1987). Methodologic problems created by variations between programs make this a difficult question (Rubin 1982). Economic analysis of the benefits of such programs is even more problematic. But a comparative cost-benefit analysis comparing the highly acclaimed comprehensive community treatment program of Madison, Wisconsin, to conventional hospitalization (with outpatient follow-up) yielded a slight advantage for the community program when patients' income from employment was taken into account (Weisbrod et al. 1980). The analysis "valued" only easily monetized costs and benefits—e.g., hospital and clinic costs, families' expenses, law enforcement costs, payments from government entitlement programs, and patients' earnings. Benefits that were difficult to monetize, like patient satisfaction and remission of clinical symptomatology, were assessed but not included in the overall, quantitative analysis. The unmonetized data heavily favored the community program.[18]

As the authors of the Wisconsin study note, the summation of monetizable costs and benefits would have yielded an advantage for conventional hospitalization had the much higher earnings of patients in the community program not been taken into account. From the fiscal perspective of the governmental units that paid for both programs, conventional hospitalization was preferable. The opposite result held from a social welfare perspective. But if the Wisconsin data roughly reflect the cost-benefit comparison between intensive community programs and conventional care more generally, the institutional capacity of government to make the *socially* preferable choice for the chronically mentally ill is in doubt, especially in view of the disabilities of the mentally ill in political competition for public resources. Nor, if community treatment superior to conventional care from a social welfare perspective is more costly to government than conventional care, would advocates of community treatment do well to promote it as cheaper. Should such advocacy succeed, its disingenuity would return to haunt. Should the advocates so com-

---

18. Counting such unmonetized costs and benefits is a more problematic enterprise than Weisbrod et al. acknowledge. Thorough discussion of the conceptual problems inherent in such a utilitarian calculus is beyond the scope of this paper. In his comments on an earlier draft of this paper, Heathcote Wales pointed out one awkward difficulty—whether (and how) such costs and benefits should be counted when experienced by third parties (e.g., persons in the community who dislike the presence of the mentally ill).

promise on the quality of community care that it becomes genuinely cheaper, they would risk giving up the social welfare advantage that makes their cause worthwhile.

Emerging professional consensus.   A developing consensus about the clinical and social needs of the chronically mentally ill in the community is evident not only in the academic literature but also in the official pronouncements of professional bodies. An American Psychiatric Association task force on the homeless mentally ill declared in 1984 that homelessness in this population is symptomatic of the nation's failure to create a comprehensive and integrated system of community care (Lamb and Talbott 1986). The task force urged that the disabled mentally ill be assured of a dependable income source, a range of community housing options graded by level of social functioning, social and occupational rehabilitation programs, family education and support, and intensive clinical services (including community outreach programs capable of anticipating crises and intervening quickly when they develop). The panel recommended that responsibility for integrating these services and entitlements for each patient be vested in a single case manager and that coordination between service agencies be vastly improved.

Such integration of clinical, rehabilitation, and support services has become a feature of some private sector programs for patients who are well insured or otherwise able to afford the costs. Moreover, although some state mental health officials persist in denying the need of chronic patients for ongoing, prophylactic outpatient contact unless they display unremitting psychiatric symptoms (Roth et al. 1986), state agencies have begun to embrace the language of the case management model. However, resource allocation and programmatic action in the public sector have lagged far behind the development of professional consensus. The gap between the emerging standard of comprehensive care and public psychiatry practice contrasts remarkably with the availability of public sector insurance and private sector cross-subsidies to support advanced *medical* services for many poor people.

In short, an emerging professional consensus well supported by empirical evidence holds that the lot of the chronically mentally ill can be substantially improved through the development of comprehensive, well-integrated community programs. The main focus of mental health policy in the 1990s ought to be closure of the gap between this consensus and current reality. Absent the political and fiscal limits that today constrain policy development, we might envision some new, large-scale federal initiative in this direction. But reform in the 1990s will probably have to occur within a restrictive framework of federal budget deficits and intensifying political competition for public resources. In this environment, the political weakness of the mentally ill will make major increases in society's commitment to them unlikely. Accordingly, to be practical, we shall offer some legislative recommendations that take account of this constraint. Before doing so, however, we shall consider the prospects for progress in the courts toward closing the gap between public psychiatry practice and the emerging professional standard of comprehensive community care.

Legal prospects.   Efforts to establish a legal basis for the imposition of minimum standards of mental health care have centered on the due process clauses of the Constitution. From the perspective of advocates for the chronically mentally ill, the results have been frustrating. Except within settings of involuntary confinement, the U.S. Supreme Court has rejected the notion that the due process clauses impose any affirmative obligation upon government to provide medical or other social services.[19] Most recently in *DeShaney v. Winnebago Co. Department of Social Services*, the court declared that substantive due process requirements "generally confer no affirmative right to governmental aid, even where such aid may be necessary to secure life, liberty, or property interests."[20] Constitutional litigation would thus appear to be an unlikely tool for transforming the care of the mentally ill in the community.

In contrast, tort doctrine may offer legal advocates for the mentally ill some room to maneuver. The principle that an actor who takes on a task, whether voluntarily or for consideration, has a duty to perform that task with reasonable care[21] has been invoked repeatedly to hold medical service providers liable in tort.[22] It furnishes a plausible doctrinal basis for holding providers of clinical services to the chronically mentally ill liable for failure to provide or arrange

---

19. The Court has held that the state is constitutionally obligated to provide involuntarily committed mental patients with clinical and other services necessary to ensure their "reasonable safety" during confinement, Youngberg v. Romeo, 457 U.S. 307 (1982). The Court has also found an Eighth Amendment duty to provide adequate medical care to prison inmates, Estelle v. Gamble, 429 U.S. 97 (1976), and a due process obligation to provide medical care to suspects in police custody who were injured while being apprehended, Revere v. Massachusetts General Hospital, 463 U.S. 239 (1983). The Court has limited the scope of these decisions by insisting that the affirmative duties they recognize arise "not from the State's knowledge of the individual's predicament or from its expressions of intent to help him, but from the limitation which it has imposed on his freedom to act on his own behalf," DeShaney v. Winnebago Co. Department of Social Services, 109 S. Ct. 998 (1989).

20. 109 S. Ct. 998 (1989) (Fourteenth Amendment due process clause imposes no state obligation to protect child from parental violence even where state agency responsible for investigating possible cases of child abuse had received a prior complaint).

21. Writing for the majority in DeShaney, Chief Justice Rehnquist suggested that this principle, incorporated into the *Restatement (Second) of Torts*, Section 323 (1965), could form the basis of a theory of state tort liability for government actors who voluntarily assume duties and then perform them negligently. The federal government has been held liable on this theory for negligent performance of protective and regulatory duties. E.g., Indian Towing v. United States, 350 U.S. 61 (1955) (action under Federal Tort Claims Act for damages to vessel that ran aground when lighthouse operated by U.S. Coast Guard negligently went out).

22. E.g., Stanturf v. Sipes, 447 S.W.2d 558 (Mo. 1969) (hospital's refusal to admit patient was actionable negligence where hospital maintained emergency service and patient presented with condition that required emergency care).

for adequate community care (Bach 1989). Plaintiffs could attempt to establish a standard of comprehensive community care by producing evidence of the developing professional consensus discussed herein. Proof of the comprehensive care provided by some private programs to patients able to pay for it and evidence of the positions taken officially by the American Psychiatric Association and other professional bodies could be presented.

However, an attempt to establish such a standard of care would face serious obstacles. Most obviously, a much less intensive level of care is commonplace, not only for indigent patients who obtain care from public facilities but also for well-insured patients able to pay for private treatment. It is true that courts have occasionally held clinical practitioners to standards of care higher than those set by customary practice,[23] on the ground that the professional customs at issue failed to meet tort law's requirement of reasonable prudence (Schwartz and Komesar 1978).[24] But the comprehensive community care discussed herein includes a broad array of services—e.g., occupational rehabilitation and case management—not traditionally conceived of as medical. Judicial reluctance to extend medical malpractice law to encompass the provision of social services would probably pose a formidable barrier to the establishment of a legal standard of comprehensive community care.

Were it to be successful, such litigation would force providers of care to the chronically mentally ill to internalize some of the costs of their failure to provide a socially optimal level of care. From a reformist perspective, the premise justifying litigation is that providers (particularly state mental health agencies, with legislative support) would respond to the disincentives of tort liability by upgrading community support and treatment services.[25]

This premise is open to serious doubt. A thorough analysis of the potential institutional impact of such litigation is beyond the scope of this paper,[26] but we will suggest several concerns. In theory, liability for losses suffered by patients due to failure to provide a socially optimal standard of community care should function as an incentive for improving that care.[27] But the frac-

---

23. E.g., Gates v. Jensen, 92 Wn.2d 246, 595 P.2d 919 (1979) (for patient with borderline eye pressure readings suggesting high risk of glaucoma, reasonable prudence required higher-than-customary standard of care).

24. Judicial willingness to do so is classically traced to Judge Learned Hand's admonition that industry custom is not in itself the measure of "reasonable prudence" and that "a whole calling may have unduly lagged in the adoption of new and available devices." The T. J. Hooper, 60 F.2d 737, 740 (2d Cir. 1932).

25. Should courts evince a willingness to intervene in the organization of services by granting injunctive relief, this aim might be achieved more directly (Bach 1989).

26. Multiple transaction cost problems are raised by the patchwork nature of responsibility for care of the indigent chronically mentally ill and the complex contractual and other relationships between state mental health agencies, private hospitals, outpatient clinics, rehabilitation programs, residential facilities, etc.

27. Note that unless a system of care is held liable for *all* losses to society (externalities) that

tured state of institutional responsibilities for community care could inhibit socially rational responses to liability. Some private clinics, unable to marshal the state or philanthropic resources necessary to meet the standard of comprehensive community care, might simply go out of business, leaving the mentally ill with less care. Likewise, private hospitals that now provide inpatient care for the indigent mentally ill but do not operate outpatient programs for these patients might respond rationally to liability for negligent discharge by reducing or eliminating such admissions. Public facilities could engage in analogous behavior. For a facility without overall, mandatory responsibility for organizing and providing services to the chronically mentally ill, cutting back on services may be a more rational response (from its fiscal perspective) than improving services.

In general, only state mental health agencies possess such overall, mandatory responsibility.[28] Thus tort actions against state-run hospitals and clinics would seem to have the best prospects for achieving socially rational results. Yet socially desirable responses by state facilities are hardly a sure thing. Rather than upgrading outpatient care, state agencies might increase hospitalization of marginal patients, figuring rationally that (1) greater custodial use of existing inpatient facilities is cheaper than development of more intensive and comprehensive outpatient programs[29] and (2) even if this violated patients' liberty interests, the cost of going into court on patients' behalf would preclude a large-scale litigation effort by patients' rights advocates. In other words, state agencies might calculate that they could remain sufficiently insulated from the social cost of increased infringement upon patients' liberty that expanded custodial care would impose less of a fiscal burden than would large-scale investment in new outpatient programs.

Alternatively, state facilities might simply decide to pay the cost of liability rather than upgrading their outpatient programs. The ability of advocates for the mentally ill to litigate on a sufficiently large scale to make state agencies liable for all or most of the social cost of substandard outpatient care seems doubtful. Thus the comparative costs (to state agencies) of meeting the standard of comprehensive community care and of actual liability for failing to do so are unlikely to accurately reflect comparative social values.

Another concern is the prospect of demoralization among clinical staff faced with tort liability for failure to maintain a standard of care that they *as*

---

result from its failure to provide care at a socially optimal level, such liability will not be a sufficient incentive to boost the standard of care all the way to a socially optimal level.

28. In theory, even state mental health agencies could "go out of business" in response to liability. As noted earlier, the U.S. Constitution has been interpreted so as not to require states to assume such "affirmative duties" as caring for the mentally ill. But such an explicit abandonment of responsibility for care of the mentally ill would seem beyond the political pale.

29. On the other hand, bureaucratic and legal barriers to the transfer of patients from acute to custodial units might inhibit this response.

individuals cannot marshal the resources to meet. Were their managers, or society as a whole, to interpret tort judgments as a stigma upon individual clinicians, demoralization problems would be greatly magnified. Moreover, stigmatization of individual professionals through tort litigation might deflect political attention from institutional inadequacies.

State legislatures could respond to tort judgments against state or private mental health facilities by enacting statutes modifying the standard of care— e.g., by instructing courts to consider the means available to a defendant when determining the standard to be applied. State legislatures could also extend the reach of sovereign immunity to bar suits against government facilities.

Legislative possibilities.   More resources are badly needed to make comprehensive community care and support available to all of the chronically mentally ill in America who are unable to purchase it from private providers. But we could make much more effective use of the entitlement programs and other public resources currently available. Given current political and fiscal constraints, legislative advocates for the chronically mentally ill ought to focus their efforts on this more modest goal.

A realistic first step would be for Congress to address the fragmentation of the entitlement streams upon which the chronically mentally ill rely. Talbott and Sharfstein (1986) urge that all entitlement streams now available to this population be aggregated into a single, federally administered Social Security plan for the mentally disabled. This program would attempt to foster development of comprehensive community care by making capitation payments to qualifying comprehensive care programs, perhaps operated by state and local mental health agencies. A less ambitious step, more sensitive to state agencies' qualms about surrendering administrative and regulatory authority to the federal government, would be development of a single administrative process by which a person could qualify as mentally disabled for the purpose of receiving federal and state entitlements. Such a process would involve a single set of disability criteria, perhaps developed jointly by federal and representative state officials. States would otherwise retain authority over the design of their own entitlement programs. State compliance with this "single track" approach to eligibility could be achieved by making it a condition for state receipt of federal dollars (e.g., block grants and Medicaid) to support the mentally ill.

Conceivably, the opportunity to reduce administrative costs could make such a "single track" approach to benefits sufficiently attractive to states to compensate for the cost in lost local autonomy. The process ought to take days or weeks, not months; speed would greatly facilitate both hospital discharge planning and outpatient crisis intervention. And by making it administratively much easier for patients in the community to maintain their economic lifelines, the process would substantially reduce a source of stress that frequently triggers psychiatric decompensation. This process could incorporate regular review provisions to make it responsive to changes in clinical status. One might even imagine several different severity gradations, each triggering a different package of entitlement benefits.

A second step could be for Congress to facilitate the combination and efficient use of entitlement streams (on patients' behalf) by comprehensive community treatment and support programs that are well designed and administered. Congress could do this by (1) empowering the U.S. Department of Health and Human Services (DHHS)—or perhaps the National Institute of Mental Health directly—to make rules with which such programs would have to comply to be eligible, and (2) giving patients who qualify for benefits via our suggested "single track" an easy-to-exercise "check-off" option to assign their entitlement streams (for a limited but renewable duration) to an eligible community treatment program. Alternatively, Congress could respond to federalism concerns by assigning state mental health agencies the task of determining the eligibility of community treatment programs to receive entitlement streams.

Yet another variation is the idea of a state or local "mental health authority"—either a government agency or a public corporation akin to statewide and regional transit or redevelopment authorities (Mechanic 1987). Such an entity could itself aggregate entitlement streams and then employ them to develop comprehensive community programs. It might either provide clinical, rehabilitation, and support services directly or contract with outside service providers (perhaps on a capitation basis), restricting itself to a coordinating and regulatory role. One might imagine the development of a heterogeneous system, with community treatment programs in some states able to accept direct assignment of individual patients' entitlement streams while in other states the process would be mediated by mental health authorities.

A further step toward facilitating the development of comprehensive community programs would be to channel available federal and state *housing* funds—e.g., HUD Section 202 dollars—into the pool of aggregated entitlements. Today, a not-for-profit firm seeking HUD Section 202 support to develop a community residential program for the mentally disabled must go through an application process that can take up to four years.[30] Whether entitlement streams are pooled at the federal or state level or by local mental health authorities, administering Section 202 and other housing dollars as part of these pools could go a long way toward simplifying and speeding this process and toward coordinating residential programs with other services.

Finally, community care has been least successful with those chronically mentally ill people who consistently reject treatment but are not sufficiently disturbed to be subject to involuntary hospitalization. An analogous pooling

---

30. Interview with Richard Silverblatt, April 1989.

of entitlement streams to create safe and supportive sheltered environments for these people, without requiring them to accept treatment, merits consideration. These residences need not be supervised by mental health professionals, but those in charge should make continuing attempts to encourage residents to accept treatment, and mental health services should be easily available. In the long run, we suspect, winning the trust of these people through such programs will go further toward engaging them in treatment than will less restrictive civil commitment laws and expanded efforts to coerce them into treatment.

Conclusion

We have offered no grand or simple design for action by government to eliminate the problems of the chronic and disabled mentally ill. Rather, we have tried to remain sensitive to the constraints imposed by other claims on public resources, by the profound psychosocial deficits of the chronically mentally ill and the limited efficacy of our best clinical methods, and by the American cultural and legal commitment to individual autonomy and the sharing of power by multiple levels of government. In so doing, we have also implicitly acknowledged a tragic reality—that the deficits and needs of the severely mentally ill do not mesh well with our culture of autonomy, pluralism, and limited state authority. We have suggested some tinkering in the interstices of these limits, in the hope of mitigating this tragedy. We are persuaded that, by tinkering, some good can be accomplished.

References

American Psychiatric Association. 1987. *Diagnostic and Statistical Manual of Mental Disorders, Third Edition, Revised*. Washington, DC: APA.

Anderson, D., D. Reiss, and G. Hogarty. 1986. *Schizophrenia in the Family: A Practitioner's Guide to Psychoeducation and Management*. New York: Guilford Press.

Arce, A., and M. Vergare. 1984. Identifying and Characterizing the Mentally Ill Among the Homeless. In *The Homeless Mentally Ill: A Task Force Report of the American Psychiatric Association*. Washington, DC: APA.

Bach, J. 1989. Requiring Due Care in the Process of Patient Deinstitutionalization: Toward a Common Law Approach to Mental Health Law Reform. *Yale Law Journal* 98: 1153–72.

Bowers, M. 1980. Biochemical Processes in Schizophrenia: An Update. *Schizophrenia Bulletin* 6: 393–403.

Braff, C., and D. Saccuzzo. 1985. The Time Course of Information-Processing Deficits in Schizophrenia. *American Journal of Psychiatry* 142: 170–74.

Braun, P., et al. 1981. Overview: Deinstitutionalization of Psychiatric Patients, a Critical Review of Outcome Studies. *American Journal of Psychiatry* 138: 736–49.

Burt, M., and K. Pittman. 1985. *Testing the Social Safety Net*. Washington, DC: Urban Institute Press.

Council of State Governments. 1950. *The Mental Health Programs of the 48 States: A Report to the Governors' Conference*. Chicago: Council of State Governments.

Cournos, F. 1987a. The Impact of Environmental Factors on Outcome in Residential Programs. *Hospital and Community Psychiatry* 38: 848–52.

————. 1987b. Hospital Outcome Studies: Implications for the Treatment of the Very Ill Patient. *Psychiatric Clinics of North America* 10: 165–76.

Dain, N. 1980. The Chronic Mental Patient in Nineteenth-Century America. *Psychiatric Annals* 10: 323–27.

Durman, E., B. Davis, and R. Bovbjerg. 1984. Block Grants and the New Federalism: The Second Year Experience. Washington, DC: The Urban Institute.

Ennis, B. 1972. *Prisoners of Psychiatry: Mental Patients, Psychiatrists, and the Law*. New York: Harcourt Brace Jovanovich.

Foley, H., and S. Sharfstein. 1983. *Madness and Government*. Washington, DC: American Psychiatric Press.

Frank, R., and L. Kessler. 1984. State Medicaid Limitations for Mental Health Services. *Hospital and Community Psychiatry* 35: 213–15.

Friedman, R. 1985. Resistance to Alternatives to Hospitalization. *Psychiatric Clinics of North America* 8: 471–82.

Gelberg, L., L. Linn, and B. Leake. 1988. Mental Health, Alcohol and Drug Use, and Criminal History Among Homeless Adults. *American Journal of Psychiatry* 145: 191–96.

Goffman, E. 1961. *Asylums*. New York: Doubleday Anchor.

Goldman, H., and A. Gattozzi. 1988. Murder in the Cathedral Revisited: President Reagan and the Mentally Disabled. *Hospital and Community Psychiatry* 39: 505–9.

Goldman, H., A. Gattozzi, and C. Taube. 1981. Defining and Counting the Chronically Mentally Ill. *Hospital and Community Psychiatry* 32: 21–27.

Greer, S., and A. Greer. 1984. The Continuity of Moral Reform: Community Mental Health Centers. *Social Science and Medicine* 19: 397–404.

Grob, G. 1983. *Mental Illness and American Society, 1875–1940*. Princeton, NJ: Princeton University Press.

Gronfein, W. 1985. Incentives and Intentions in Mental Health Policy: A Comparison of the Medicaid and Community Mental Health Programs. *Journal of Health and Social Behavior* 26: 192–206.

Hersch, C. 1972. Social History, Mental Health, and Community Control. *American Psychologist* 27: 44.

Jerrell, J., and J. Larsen. 1984. Policy Shifts and Organizational Adaptation: A Review of Current Developments. *Community Mental Health Journal* 20: 282–93.

Keogel, P., A. Burnam, and R. Farr. 1988. The Prevalence of Specific Psychiatric Disorders Among Homeless Individuals in the Inner City of Los Angeles. *Archives of General Psychiatry* 45: 1085–92.

Kiesler, C., and A. Sibulkin. 1987. *Mental Hospitalization: Myths and Facts About a National Crisis*. Newbury Park, CA: Sage.

Lamb, R., and M. Mills. 1986. Needed Changes in Law and Procedure for the Chronically Mentally Ill. *Hospital and Community Psychiatry* 37: 475–80.

Lamb, R., and J. Talbott. 1986. The Homeless Mentally Ill: The Perspective of the American Psychiatric Association. *Journal of the American Medical Association* 256: 498–501.

Larsen, J. 1987. Community Mental Health Services in Transition. *Community Mental Health Journal* 23: 16–25.

Lehman, A. 1989. Strategies for Improving Services for the Chronic Mentally Ill. *Hospital and Community Psychiatry* 40: 916–20.

Lerman, P. 1985. Deinstitutionalization and Welfare Policies. *Annals of the American Academy of Political and Social Science* 419: 132–55.

Marmor, T., and K. Gill. 1986. The Political and Economic Context of Mental Health Care in the United States (unpublished manuscript).

Mechanic, D. 1985. Mental Health and Social Policy: Initiatives for the 1980s. *Health Affairs* 4: 75–88.

———. 1987. Correcting Misconceptions in Mental Health Policy. *Milbank Quarterly* 65: 203–30.

Milbank Memorial Fund. 1962. *Decentralization of Psychiatric Services and Continuity of Care*. New York: Milbank Memorial Fund.

Morrissey, J., and H. Goldman. 1984. Cycles of Reform in the Care of the Chronically Mentally Ill. *Hospital and Community Psychiatry* 35: 785–93.

———. 1986. Care and Treatment of the Mentally Ill in the United States. *Annals of the American Academy of Political and Social Science* 484: 12–27.

Moynihan, D. P. 1986. *Family and Nation*. New York: Harcourt Brace Jovanovich.

Okin, R. 1983. The Future of State Hospitals: Should There Be One? *American Journal of Psychiatry* 140: 577–81.

Rochefort, D. 1984. Origins of the "Third Psychiatric Revolution": The Community Mental Health Centers Act of 1963. *Journal of Health Policy, Politics and Law* 9: 1–30.

Ropers, R. 1988. *The Invisible Homeless*. New York: Human Sciences Press.

Roth, D., G. Bean, and P. Hyde. 1986. Homelessness and Mental Health Policy: Developing an Appropriate Role for the 1980s. *Community Mental Health Journal* 22: 203–14.

Rothman, D. 1971. *Discovery of the Asylum*. Boston: Little, Brown.

———. 1980. *Conscience and Convenience*. Boston: Little, Brown.

Rubin, J. 1982. Cost Measurement and Cost Data in Mental Health Settings. *Hospital and Community Psychiatry* 33: 750–54.

Schmidt, L., A. Reinhardt, R. Kane, and D. Olsen. 1977. The Mentally Ill in Nursing Homes: New Back Wards in the Community. *Archives of General Psychiatry* 34: 687–91.

Schussheim, H. 1989. A Sanctuary Worth Saving. *Washington Post*, 8 October, p. C4.

Schwartz, W., and N. Komesar. 1978. Damages and Deterrence: An Economic View of Medical Malpractice. *New England Journal of Medicine* 298: 1282–87.

Scull, A. 1985. Deinstitutionalization and Public Policy. *Social Science and Medicine* 20: 545–52.

Segal, S., and O. Aviram. 1978. *The Mentally Ill in Community-Based Sheltered Care: A Study of Community Care and Social Integration*. New York: Wiley.

Shadish, W., and R. Bootzin. 1984. Nursing Homes: The New Total Institution in Mental Health Policy. *International Journal of Partial Hospitalization* 2: 251–62.

Starr, P. 1982. *The Social Transformation of American Medicine*. New York: Basic Books.

Szasz, T. 1963. *Law, Liberty, and Psychiatry: An Inquiry into the Social Uses of Mental Health Practices*. New York: Macmillan.

Talbott, J., and S. Sharfstein. 1986. A Proposal for Future Funding of Chronic and Episodic Mental Illness. *Hospital and Community Psychiatry* 37: 1126–30.

Test, M., and L. Stein. 1978. Community Treatment of the Chronic Patient: Research Overview. *Schizophrenia Bulletin* 4: 350–64.

Tsuang, M., and R. Vandermey. 1980. *Genes and the Mind: Inheritance of Mental Illness*. New York: Oxford University Press.

U.S. Bureau of the Census. 1983. *Statistical Abstract of the United States*. Washington, DC: Government Printing Office.

U.S. Department of Health and Human Services, Steering Committee on the Chronically Mentally Ill. 1980. *Toward a National Plan for the Chronically Mentally Ill*. Washington, DC: DHHS.

Usdin, G. 1980. Preface. In *The Family: Evaluation and Treatment*, ed. C. Hofling and J. Lewis. New York: Brunner Mazel.

Vaughn, C., and J. Leff. 1976. The Influence of Family and Social Factors on the Course of Psychiatric Illness. *British Journal of Psychiatry* 129: 125–37.

Weinberger, D., E. Torrey, and N. Neophytides. 1979. Lateral Cerebral Ventricular Enlargement in Chronic Schizophrenia. *Archives of General Psychiatry* 36: 735–39.

Weisbrod, B., M. Test, and L. Stein. 1980. Alternative to Mental Hospitalization: Economic Cost-Benefit Analysis. *Archives of General Psychiatry* 37: 400–405.

Wilkinson, C. 1983. Mental Health Policy and the Political Process. *American Journal of Psychiatry* 140: 875–76.

Zusman, J. 1975. The Philosophic Basis for a Community and Social Psychiatry. In *An Assessment of the Community Mental Health Movement*, ed. W. E. Barton and C. J. Sanborn. Lexington, MA: D. C. Heath.

The Medically Uninsured: Problems, Policies, and Politics

Lawrence D. Brown

Abstract. The ranks of the medically uninsured have grown significantly in recent years, but no consensus on a policy solution has emerged. After summarizing the characteristics of the uninsured population, this paper reviews diverse policy responses and their troubled political prospects.

The United States has the disturbing distinction that it, alone among Western democracies, permits a sizable percentage of its population to go entirely without health insurance coverage. Over the 1980s both the scope of the problem and national attention to it grew substantially. In the early 1990s, however, no solution appears to be imminent or even dimly visible on the horizon. This paper begins with an overview of the nature of the problem, proceeds to examine the major policy options now under discussion, and concludes with an account of the political forces that may—or may not—generate action.

Who are the uninsured?

Depending on one's preferred data set, between 31 million and 37 million Americans, or between 12.9 percent and 17.6 percent of the nonaged population, have no health insurance.[1] The problem worsened over the 1980s. The most widely cited estimates indicate that in 1977, 26.2 million people (13.8 percent of the nonaged population) had no insurance. By 1980 the number had grown to 28.6 million (14.6 percent), by 1983 to 32 million (16.1 percent), and by 1986 to 36.8 million (Butler 1988: 9). One-third of the uninsured are less than 18 years old, and another third are between the ages of

The author is grateful to Rhonda Davis Poirier for research assistance and to the Robert Wood Johnson Foundation for support for the evaluation (of its Health Program for the Uninsured) on which this article draws heavily.

1. On the lower estimate (for 1987), see Moyer (1989). For the higher figure (for 1986), see Butler (1988).

18 and 24 (Short 1989: 5–6). More than one-third (35.7 percent) of uninsured children are in families with earnings below the poverty line (Chollet 1988).

Contrary to casual impression, lack of health insurance is more a problem among the nonpoor than the poor. In 1986 three in ten uninsured people lived in families below the federal poverty line, though nearly half fell below 150 percent of it (Congressional Research Service 1988: 170),[2] and more of these uninsured were employed than unemployed. In 1980, 55.6 percent of those without insurance were working—38.7 percent full time, 16.9 percent part time (Monheit et al. 1985: 349). Another 22.3 percent were dependents of uninsured employees, and 10–12 percent more were uninsured dependents of insured employees. In sum, 87–89 percent of the medically uninsured have some relation to the workplace (Butler 1988: 14).[3] Within the workplace, lack of insurance varies strongly and inversely with income. In 1986 about 15 percent of workers without insurance from their jobs earned more than $25,000 per year; the figure rose to 22.7 percent for incomes between $15,000 and $20,000, to 36.5 percent between $10,000 and $15,000, to 62.2 percent between $5,000 and $10,000, and to 88.6 percent below $5,000 (Congressional Research Service 1988: 164). Three-fourths of the working uninsured earn under $10,000 annually (U.S. GAO 1989: 20). The strong correlation between low earnings and lack of insurance argues against defining solutions entirely in terms of work-related coverage, for even as the erosion of Medicaid eligibility for the working poor over the 1980s has aggravated the problem, expansions of the program in the 1990s could help to alleviate it.

Insurance status varies with type of firm. Industries in which 50 percent or more of workers lacked health insurance related to their own jobs in 1986 include farming, forestry, personal services, entertainment and recreation, retail trade, business and repair services, and construction (Congressional Research Service 1988: 165). Insurance status also varies with size of firm: In general, the smaller the firm, the less likely that it offers health coverage to its workers. In 1983, about 63 percent of firms with fewer than 25 employees offered no insurance; only 20.5 percent of firms with 500–999 workers and 14.6 percent of those with 1,000 workers or more offered none (ibid.: 166). In 1987, 92 percent of firms without employee health plans had fewer than 10 employees (AHA 1988: 20, 101). It would be a mistake, however, to overstate the connection between lack of insurance and being employed in a small business. One analysis of 1984 data found that slightly fewer than half

---

2. An estimate by the GAO found that 38.5 percent of the population below the poverty line was uninsured (U.S. GAO 1989: 19).

3. The GAO found that only 14 percent of the uninsured lived in families whose head "neither worked nor sought work at any time during the year" (U.S. GAO 1989: 18).

(48 percent) of uninsured workers and their families were attached to firms with a workforce of 1–24 people. About one-fourth (26 percent) were in firms with 500 workers or more, while 15 percent were in firms with 25–99 employees, and 12 percent were in firms with 100–499 workers (ibid.: 20–22).

The availability of employee health plans varies not only with industry size and type, but also with larger economic trends whose effects are imperfectly understood. It is often argued that shifts from manufacturing to service jobs and from full-time to part-time employment have increased the ranks of the uninsured and will continue to do so. Others contend that the percent of the nonaged population covered by health insurance accompanying their own job increased slightly between 1979 and 1986, but that these gains were offset by "the most dramatic trend," namely, "the decline in the percent of the non-elderly population covered by employment-based plans through another family member." (Such coverage fell from 34.3 percent to 31.4 percent; Congressional Research Service 1988: 181–87.) As the price of health insurance has risen, some employers have economized by eliminating family coverage or reducing their contributions towards its purchase. Between 1977 and 1983, two-thirds of employers paid the full cost of enrollee coverage and 40 percent met the full cost of covering dependents. By 1987, these figures had fallen to 57 percent and about one-third of employers, respectively (ibid: 110). These trends suggest that the problems of the uninsured are closely linked to larger issues of health care cost containment. Rising health insurance premiums may fall with special severity on small firms, because, it is argued, "when it comes to family coverage, there is a very strong *negative* correlation between the size of the group and the employer's premium share" (AHA 1988: 46). That is, those small employers who do offer such coverage are less likely than larger ones to require significant employee contributions. When hard-pressed small firms face rapidly rising premiums, they may be especially tempted to drop health insurance altogether, eliminate dependent coverage, or increase employee contributions beyond what lower-income workers can afford.

Finally, although the evidence is far from iron-clad, some data suggest that lack of insurance has a discernible negative impact on access to care. Studies have found that on average, the uninsured see doctors only two-thirds as often as the insured (the low-income uninsured average only about half as many doctor visits as the low-income insured), make more use of emergency rooms and hospital outpatient departments, and spend only three-quarters as many days in the hospital (though uninsured children use more inpatient days then do those with insurance) (Congressional Research Service 1988: 225–42). A 1986 survey found that about 20 million Americans reported that they had met financial barriers in their efforts to get care, and over one million declared that they had tried but failed to get care because of cost (Robert Wood Johnson Foundation 1987).

What can be done?

In principle, the problem of the medically uninsured is amenable to a straight-forward solution, one that is (as Ronald Reagan liked to say) simple, though not easy. The United States could emulate its Western democratic peers by enacting a program of national health insurance with universal entitlements and uniform benefits. Reluctant as ever to incorporate policy entitlements within the sphere of citizenship rights, the nation has rejected this course and may well continue to do so. Nor is there much immediate prospect of federal leadership. Throughout the 1980s the Reagan administration insisted that the uninsured were not a federal problem, that the huge federal budget deficit precluded initiatives on their behalf, and that their plight ought to be taken as a bracing challenge to the states. By federal default, then, policymaking has been largely a catalogue of fits and starts among the fifty states. The most prominent[4] programmatic components may be summarized as the "four Ms"—markets, mandates, Medicaid, and miscellaneous.

Markets.   One strategy calls for the development of new insurance products that will be readily marketable—meaning both acceptable and affordable— to firms that do not now insure their workers. This approach has some strong a priori appeals. The U.S. system relies very heavily on employment-based insurance for most of its nonaged population and, for most of that population, the system works, albeit unevenly. Most of the uninsured either work or are dependents of workers. And this line of attack appeals to the innate intuitions of U.S. policymakers, who are always inclined to exhaust the market first, calling in government only as a last resort in response to demonstrated market failure. Surely, then, America's fabled ingenuity in product design, organizational innovation, and marketing expertise can bring the system close to universal coverage.[5]

Variations on the market approach are now being tested here and there, most prominently in 15 sites supported by the Health Program for the Un-insured, launched by the Robert Wood Johnson Foundation in 1985. This writer, in collaboration with Catherine McLaughlin of the University of Michigan, is now evaluating the program; a fair assessment of outcomes remains at least two years off. The ups and downs of the sites to date, however, suggest that market-building faces many more practical problems than readily meet

---

4. Here "most prominent" means proposals that stand fairly high on the agendas of a sizable number of states. This excludes from discussion various options that are intellectually important but (so far) of limited practical weight (for instance, universal insurance by means of managed competition) or that may have exhausted their fifteen minutes of fame in the policy process (for example, state health insurance pools). On managed competition, see Enthoven and Kronick (1989). On pools, see Bovbjerg and Koller (1986).

5. For a good overview, see Bovbjerg (1986).

the theoretical eye. Indeed, an interim evaluation might be summarized with the rhetorical challenge: "If you're so smart, why ain't you rich?"

As is so often the case with market schemes, the supposedly straightforward economic dynamics of new insurance products become enmeshed in coalition-building challenges deriving from the discordant interests of multiple groups. The Johnson sites suggest that getting the strategy off the ground—to say nothing of making it succeed—demands the cooperation of six distinct groups.

First, because the elements of new insurance products do not spring out of thin air, a sponsor is needed to assess local markets (employers, employees, insurers, providers) and to recruit an insurer to take the lead in further development of the product. In the Johnson program local staffs (funded by the foundation) played this role, which might otherwise have fallen outside the mission or resources of community organizations.

Second, employers (who must usually make a significant financial contribution to new coverage) must be informed of, and persuaded to buy, the new product. But small businessmen often prove to be a hard sell. Many complain that they live on the financial edge and risk being pushed over it by the costs of new insurance. Most lack benefit managers or other specialized assistance in pondering, weighing, and administering health insurance. A few are ideologically averse to such "fringe" benefits.

Third, employees themselves must be convinced that a new insurance offering is a good buy. Although when polled, workers enthusiastically declare their general desire for coverage, getting them to sign on the bottom line can be another matter. "Young immortals" with little concern for risk may prefer to save their money and take their chances. Some cynics are content to let "the system" cover the costs if they get sick. Many want insurance but face more pressing claims on their low incomes, such as housing and food. Others want insurance but have unrealistic expectations, demanding comprehensive coverage for small premium contributions. When costs are to be borne entirely by employers and workers, the gap between acceptability and affordability may be unbridgeable.

Fourth, marketing a plan presupposes that an insurer has agreed to develop and endorse it. Some insurers decline to write policies for small groups (or limit their small group business) because they fear the utilization and cost liabilities of such groups. Those that do work this market tend to underwrite heavily, screen risks carefully, and keep a close eye on profits, dropping groups (and sometimes their entire small group line) if returns fall too low. Rates may rise rapidly from year to year, reflecting fluctuations in utilization or losses elsewhere in their health (and other) lines; this encourages "churning" (shifting of firms among insurers in search of a better deal) and costs some workers and dependents their coverage. The uneven progress of the Johnson projects spotlights the basic tension between the mission of insurance as an *institution*, which supposedly exists to spread, pool, and manage risk, and insurance as an *industry*, a set of firms bent on spotting, shirking, and shifting risk.

Having agreed to develop innovative insurance offerings, most of the local Johnson staffs soon recognized that they had little idea how to proceed. Most turned, understandably, to their community-serving Blue Cross plans, which generally offered them warm smiles, firm handshakes, and heartfelt regrets that the Blues' deep practical insights and deeper fiscal deficits argued against involvement in chancy ventures at that time.[6] The local staffs then began canvassing lists of commercial firms, mostly small and little known, who were rumored to be seeking experience with, or solid footing on the ground floor in, the small business market. Identifying a suitable insurer and then resolving disagreements on dozens of items of mutual interest (including underwriting rules) took months and much delayed the progress of the projects.

Fifth, new insurance benefits mean little unless providers are available to deliver care. Determined to keep coverage affordable by holding the line on costs, most projects have put their bets on "managed care," usually meaning, among other things, delimited service sites and gatekeeping primary care physicians. Those who staff such systems, however, often fear that they will be asked to crowd their schedules and facilities with many new patients whose care is remunerated at deeply discounted rates. Hospitals and physicians already delivering much uncompensated care may be willing to take fifty cents on the dollar for some old and new patients, but "mainstream" providers may balk. Meanwhile, workers newly reaching into their wallets to pay for health insurance may insist on visiting mainstream providers and may resist sharing waiting rooms with Medicaid types, whose care is also being managed to contain costs.

Given these difficulties, it is a plausible (though unproven) hypothesis that new market offerings financed entirely by small businessmen and lower-income workers will frequently fail to bridge the gap between affordability and acceptability. Quite possibly, then, a "pure" market strategy can be salvaged only by inviting in, sixth, that impurest of partners, government, to share (and perhaps help control) costs. Government subsidies, which reduce direct costs to employers and workers, may make an acceptable product affordable. But such subsidies raise a host of perplexing policy questions. How large will the subsidies be? For how many firms and workers? Extended on what terms? For

---

6. This is not to say that Blue Cross's reluctance in the Johnson projects is necessarily generalizable to all or most Blue plans. For example, in January 1990 Blue Cross of Western Pennsylvania announced "Special Care," a new program unrelated to the Johnson efforts that will offer subsidized coverage to as many as 20,000 people in 29 counties. For other innovations by Blue Cross and Blue Shield, see Freudenheim (1990).

how long? Subject to what cost constraints? These, of course, are precisely the public policy issues the market approach was expected to circumvent.

Mandates.   Considering the many tribulations that attend creative uses of the insurance market to assist the uninsured, some contend that mandating is a more equitable and direct approach. *Mandating* in this context means public law(s) ordering employers to provide insurance benefits (variously defined) to all or some of their workers on pain of penalty (a tax surcharge, say) should they fail. Mandating proposals are not new: in the early 1970s, for example, they were a basic element in the Nixon administration's National Health Insurance Standards plan, then much derided by liberals such as Democratic senator Edward Kennedy of Massachusetts, who later reevaluated and endorsed the approach in the darker days of Reaganomics. While the Congress debates the merits of mandating, it has, however, checkmated states that might meanwhile choose to enact their own versions. Section 514 of the Employment Retirement and Income Security Act (ERISA) of 1974 permits states to regulate insurance companies but exempts from their reach employers' benefit plans, which means that states cannot, strictly speaking, "mandate" that employers offer health insurance. Those committed to doing so—notably Hawaii, whose mandating law of 1974 was abruptly invalidated by ERISA— must seek a federal waiver, which, as Hawaii's efforts showed, is not easily won (Fox and Schaffer 1989). Though often called "mandating," the Health Security Act adopted in Massachusetts in 1988 in fact seeks to skirt the ERISA preemption by declining to dictate the contents of employer coverage. The law says in essence that employers can avoid a surcharge on their payroll taxes by buying each eligible worker a health insurance policy worth $1,680.

Although in theory mandating avoids the contingencies of the market approach, in practice staying on the right side of ERISA creates many of the same problems now faced by the Johnson sites. Massachusetts businessmen "mandated" by the law now bear an obligation that many do not know how to fulfill, and so the state (especially the Department of Medical Security, created to implement the new law) must educate them about the nature and extent of their duties, help them identify and contract with suitable insurance plans, and worry about how escalating costs and premiums will be addressed once the law goes into effect. A serious state budget deficit and battling between the Dukakis administration and the state's hospitals did nothing to ease implementation.

Some advocates of mandating believe that it is both fair and feasible. Most firms—even many small ones—do offer coverage to their workers; mandating merely levels the playing field by forbidding free riders to dodge responsibility and shift costs to others. Critics reply that employers who fail to offer insurance do so not because they want to but because financial realities tie their hands. Faced with a mandate, such economic unfortunates will go out of business, lay off workers, reduce full-time workers to part time, forego wage increases, or combine these adaptations.[7] No one knows how seriously to take such predictions, but states bent on preserving their reputations for offering a good business climate—which includes most states—are fearful of the symbolic signals that a thorough public debate might transmit.

Other critics point out that mandating per se does nothing to constrain costs and therefore does nothing to assure the continuing affordability of the insurance it requires employers to provide. Sensitive to this problem (often described as the Achilles' heel of the Massachusetts plan, which leaves the dominant financing and delivery systems largely intact), the New York State Department of Health has proposed that its plan for universal access (UNI*CARE) balances its employer mandates and public subsidies with a Single Payer Authority with comprehensive rate-setting powers. The plan's admirable conceptual coherence, however, carries the price of concentrating the political opposition of employers, private insurers, providers, and others, and the full scheme has yet to win formal endorsement from Governor Mario Cuomo.

Medicaid. Insofar as marketing and mandating strategies fail to work, expanding Medicaid may be an appealing policy alternative. It is the only available vehicle for the unemployed uninsured and a potentially important one for low-income uninsured workers now excluded by federal and state cutbacks that have left about 60 percent of the poor ineligible for the program. In recent years Congress has adopted various measures, some requiring and others permitting the states to expand Medicaid eligibility and benefits, mainly for poor mothers and children, and many states have moved on their own to bring some uninsured citizens newly under Medicaid protection.[8] Because the approach does not require the development of new insurance offerings or new legislative mandates, but builds instead on an established program, it appears to be more straightforward and more amenable to the familiar politics of incremental expansion than do the aforementioned options.

Thorpe and his colleagues (1989) estimate that the 10.9 million uninsured poor could be brought under current Medicaid coverage at a public cost of about $9 billion, $5 billion federal and the rest state and local. Nine billion dollars is hardly an exorbitant sum; nonetheless, as a national strategy for the uninsured, the expansion of Medicaid presents a dilemma. Some state legislators view the program with suspicion notwithstanding its federal contribution "because its myriad requirements impede state flexibility and its open-

---

7. See, for example, the pessimistic predictions of small business respondents in the survey published by the National Federation of Independent Business in July 1989, summarized in Medical Benefits (1989).

8. For an overview, see Intergovernmental Health Policy Project (1988).

ended 'entitlement' nature impedes budget control" (Butler 1985: 230). The states with the most extensive and expensive programs have, at least in theory, the resources to enlarge them, but in many cases they have also exhausted their fiscal and political patience with Medicaid. Growing rapidly and annually threatening to unbalance the budget, the program is not viewed as a sympathetic claimant on the sizable new revenues that would be needed to extend it to many of the uninsured. Conversely, many states with relatively poor and weak programs have the will to enlarge it but lack the budgetary resources to do so and the political audacity to raise taxes for this purpose. Knowing that they can trigger generous (perhaps 70 percent) federal matching shares if they raise their own share, such states have considered various fund-raising schemes. "Sin" taxes earmarked for indigent care apparently hold limited appeal (Hospitals 1989). Confronting a narrow range of controversial options, some states have entertained "revenue assessments" on hospitals— legislation that captures a fraction of the revenues of most hospitals and pools these receipts as the state contribution to Medicaid expansions underwritten largely with federal dollars. Florida was the first state to impose such an assessment, in 1984 (Jones 1989); South Carolina and West Virginia followed suit, and others have pondered the possibility.

The main political obstacle to the strategy is, unsurprisingly, the opposition of the hospitals, which have denounced such assessments as a "sick tax" that inequitably puts the burden of enlarged insurance coverage on the backs of paying hospital patients. The assessment strategy seems to succeed when two conditions are met: first, governors (and often key health legislators) must be determined to lift their states out of the bottom quintiles on measures of breadth of Medicaid coverage and benefits and devote political capital to finding the money to do so. Such "modernizing moderates" are increasingly common in southern and other statehouses. Second, the strategy gets a boost when a state's hospitals are internally divided. In Florida, nonprofit and municipal hospitals resented the for-profits' alleged shirking of their fair share of uncompensated care and viewed the revenue assessment as a means of leveling the playing field. In South Carolina hospitals were abashed by bad publicity about real and threatened economic "dumping" of uncovered patients. The two conditions rarely converge, however, which leaves most states grumbling about federal meddling in Medicaid, little inclined to put new general revenues of their own into the program, and unwilling to battle the hospitals over "sick taxes." The fiscal and political liabilities of Medicaid as a vehicle of assistance for the non-elderly poor have become so numerous and grave that the program can probably make no more than a marginal contribution to covering the uninsured.

Miscellaneous.   Even if markets, mandates, and Medicaid worked reasonably well as solutions for the uninsured, enough citizens would probably fall between the programmatic cracks to justify the continuation (or creation) of bad debt and charity care pools, uncompensated care trust funds, and the like, which use ratesetting and other state-run mechanisms to subsidize hospitals hit hardest by losses on the uncovered. Although many analysts agree that subsidies are best directed mainly to individuals, not institutions (e.g., Blendon 1986), new benefits vested in the former are unlikely entirely to eliminate the need for continued assistance to the latter.

Is change imminent?

Policymaking based on permutations and combinations of four (or more, or fewer) uphill strategies in each (or some) of the fifty states hardly promises effectiveness or efficiency. As one ponders the fragmentation and frustration encumbering new coverage for about 15 percent of the population, one wonders when the nation will finally get on with it and embrace a national answer (whether "national health insurance" or that rose by another name) for a major national problem. Almost everyone agrees that the lingering, worsening problems of the uninsured do the nation no credit, and even conservative theorists enamored of private-sector stratagems for cost containment generally accept that the state has an important role to play in extending coverage to the uninsured. Nor can one explain inaction by invoking the old image of a politics of policy deadlocked and stalemated by structural fragmentation and the power of special interests. In the health cost-containment arena, the federal government was highly active and innovative in the 1970s and 1980s and has not feared to face down powerful groups when it saw a chance to slow the growth of its own budgetary burdens. The question about the uninsured, then, is, When, if ever, will we find the will that finds the way?

One school of thought contends that the nation's inability to solve the problem of the uninsured is a natural (albeit morbid) expression of the distinctive U.S. value system. "Are Americans really as mean as they look?" asked Uwe Reinhardt (1984) in the pointed subtitle of an insightful essay on the uninsured. To be sure, the American allegiance to economic individualism and our moralistic, punitive stance towards the poor set us apart from Europe, Canada, and other nations where solidarism is stronger and the "right" to health care is accepted as a kind of civic axiom. But "meanness" is a highly complex cultural concept. Polls indicate that Americans generally do not think it right that fellow citizens should lack care because they cannot afford it.[9] If we do not follow the argument to the new governmental entitlements to which it would seem to lead, this may be because the public wrongly believes that existing programs such as Medicaid do or could cover most of the poor,

---

9. An SRI Gallup survey is summarized in Hospitals (1987); see also Gabel et al. (1989).

fails to recognize the imperfect correlation between work and insurance, or assumes that anyone who falls seriously ill can go to the emergency room of the local hospital and get reasonable care in a timely fashion. Americans may tolerate rationing medical care by price only because we believe that it breaks down in cases of true need—a belief that even today probably remains largely accurate. Intuitively, public opinion may be saying that it prefers more red ink for providers to new red tape from government. Viewed in this context, the political problem is less the American value system than the way we fit facts to our values.

There is minor empirical support for this interpretation. In the mid-1980s some hospitals began to experiment with "dumping" as an answer to their costs of uncompensated care; in several cases, sick or wounded patients who lacked insurance were denied admission and sent, or told to go, elsewhere. Local and national media quickly jumped on these scandals and made them front-page, prime-time news. Congress sensed the rising indignation and responded quickly by forbidding economic dumping in the Consolidated Omnibus Budget Reconciliation Act of 1985.

It is very difficult, however, to move beyond episodic bursts of social conscience broadcast by the media to a lucid, sustained public understanding of the economic forces eroding the old "anyone can get care if he/she really needs it" failsafe. That, and how, impinging forces of competition and regulation visit severe penalties on providers and payers who cross-subsidize extensively between paying and nonpaying patients are not "items" among the news the media generally see fit to print, and even if they were, doleful depictions of trends in hospital accounting and budgeting probably lack sufficient melodrama to fuel a popular movement for reform. A public mood supportive of new benefits for the uninsured may be necessary to generate political action, but sufficiency probably lies in the commitment of various elites.

One such elite is big business. Corporate America bears a large share of the continually rising health care costs and has been protesting for over a decade that it finds them insupportable. Firms that ante up to insure their own workers increasingly resent financing uncompensated care delivered to workers whose employers decline to make similar provisions. In short, the ranks of the business community are split; the support of big business for reform could both engage the attention of politicians and neutralize the opposition of small business.

Providers, too, may help build the case for change. Some voluntary and public hospitals lose sizable sums on uncompensated care and, as noted above, their ability to recoup by shifting costs to paying customers is eroding (though not of course uniformly) under the pressures of competition and regulation. Opening their arms to the uninsured is bad economics, but closing them means bad publicity and a sour conscience. Physicians warned by hospital administrators to admit the uninsured only as a last resort may be shocked by the crude intrusion of economic imperatives into professional judgment, and even the more conservative among them increasingly wonder whether governmental intervention might not be a necessary evil. Business and providers could exert important influence at the state level. And these groups plus governors and other prominent state officials could apply pressure for a federal response.

Though such a coalition would indeed seem to advance the interests of its component groups, its consolidation is no sure thing. Working assertively in political concert on behalf of the uninsured would oblige business and providers to overcome their ingrained suspicions of both government and each other. And even if they did so, it is unlikely that new coverage for the uninsured would stand at the top of the agendas of the coalition's various components. The coalition for change is now, and will probably remain, wide but neither intense nor deep.

Even if a broad, committed combination of political forces unequivocally demanded governmental solutions for the uninsured, however, policymaking might degenerate into a replay of the painful politics of national health insurance. After all, 15 percent of the population now lacks health benefits because "the system" has never managed to agree on an acceptable version of universal coverage.

In progressive circles there is little doubt that the blame for the intermittent, botched attempts to create national health insurance falls on the narrow self-interest of the powerful providers and insurers who would be discomfited or displaced by change. This explanation is, at the very least, incomplete. Canada and most European nations faced skeptical or opposed providers and insurers in their debates over national health insurance, but proceeded to enact it anyway. There the *proponents* reached agreement on what to do and united behind concrete legislation. In the United States, by contrast, proponents have repeatedly split over the relative merits of cradle-to-grave "health security" coverage, catastrophic insurance, consumer choice health plans, variants on employer mandates, child care, and more.

American coalition-building politics differ structurally as well as ideologically from those of Western peers. Canadian and European advocates did not unite successfully around reforms because the rough edges of disagreement spontaneously fell away. Britain, for example, harbored deep, continuing differences between those who viewed national health insurance mainly as a form of income support and those who saw it as a means of achieving a more rational organization of the medical care system (Fox 1986). But in Britain and other European nations, disagreements were fought out within governmental structures—especially the party or the ruling coalition—that obliged proponents to sit at a bargaining table behind a closed door, fight it out in private, reach an agreement, and then emerge to defend and enact it as "the government's" program. The United States lacks such agreement-forcing structures; here the president proposes (if perchance he chooses to) and Congress disposes—often by shredding his initiative and then starting over with a dozen or two others generated by its own members. Latter-day tendencies toward divided government (for most of the last two decades Republicans have controlled the White House, Democrats the Congress) and diffusion of legislative leadership have aggravated these familiar structural features. These peculiar American characteristics of the proponents of change are at least as important in accounting for the failures of national health insurance as is the obdurate opposition of entrenched interests. In the United States debates can drag on for decades as splits among policy "leaders" remain unresolved, as opponents exploit divisions on the other side, and as windows of opportunity open briefly and in vain and then shut again. In a sense, then, the number of groups that want change, and how badly they want it, are secondary issues in coalition building. What matters most (or at any rate first) is getting a range of groups to agree on one detailed legislative agenda and then ensuring that they pledge allegiance to it and see it through. Today there is little in the politics of the uninsured that seems to signal a break with the self-indulgent, self-defeating politics of national health insurance.

Conclusions

Major policy change in the United States usually presupposes the fulfillment and convergence of three conditions. First, there must be a call to arms, a widespread sense among policy leaders that an urgent (not merely ominous or impending) social problem cries out for solution. Second, policymakers must conclude that the usual ports of first call—the market, the voluntary sector, and the professions—are not up to the job and that a governmental role in problem solving is necessary. Third, policymakers must agree on a strategic model that promises to achieve desired goals without generating unacceptable side effects. Action may fail for any or all of these three reasons— because the problem at hand is not grave enough, because the market (or other nongovernmental sectors) are thought to be plausible problem-solving instruments, or because policymakers, though prepared and committed to act, cannot decide what it makes sense to do.

In the politics of the uninsured, these three conditions have not converged. Indeed, none of the three now comes close to being met. The call to arms is muted by popular conviction that those in medical need will somehow get charitable care, by popular ignorance of the changing realities of hospital economics, and by ambivalence among business and provider groups about cooperation with government. The depletion of nongovernmental alternatives is arrested by the hope that the work-based health insurance schemes that now cover most of the population can somehow be made to embrace segments they now shun (or that shun them). Consensus on a strategic model, and coalition building around it, are impeded by the usual proliferation of preferred solutions and the absence of structural mechanisms that would discourage proponents from falling out among themselves if a political window of opportunity were to open.

References

American Hospital Association. 1988. *Promoting Health Insurance in the Workplace: State and Local Initiatives to Increase Private Coverage*. Chicago: AHA.

Blendon, Robert J., et al. 1986. Uncompensated Care by Hospitals or Public Insurance for the Poor: Does It Make a Difference? *New England Journal of Medicine* 314: 1160–63.

Bovbjerg, Randall R. 1986. Insuring the Uninsured through Private Actions. *Inquiry* 23 (Winter): 403–18.

Bovbjerg, Randall R., and Christopher F. Koller. 1986. State Health Insurance Pools: Current Performance, Future Prospects. *Inquiry* 23 (Summer): 111–21.

Butler, Patricia A. 1985. New Initiatives in Financing and Delivering Health Care for the Medically Indigent: Report on a Conference. *Law, Medicine and Health Care* 13: 230.

―――. 1988. *Too Poor to Be Sick: Access to Medical Care for the Uninsured*. Washington, DC: American Public Health Association.

Chollet, Deborah. 1988. Uninsured in the United States: The Non-Elderly Population Without Health Insurance, 1986. Washington, DC: Employee Benefit Research Institute.

Congressional Research Service. 1988. *Health Insurance and the Uninsured: Background Data and Analysis*. Washington, DC: CRS.

Enthoven, Alain, and Richard Kronick. 1989. A Consumer-Choice Health Plan for the 1990s: Universal Health Insurance in a System Designed to Promote Quality and Economy. *New England Journal of Medicine* 320: 29–37, 94–101.

Fox, Daniel M. 1986. *Health Policies, Health Politics: The British and American Experience, 1911–1965*. Princeton, NJ: Princeton University Press.

Fox, Daniel M., and Daniel C. Schaffer. 1989. Health Policy and ERISA: Interest Groups and Semipreemption. *Journal of Health Politics, Policy and Law* 14: 239–60.

Freudenheim, M. 1990. Business and Health: Insurers Testing Basic Coverage. *New York Times*, 27 March, p. D2.

Gabel, Jon, et al. 1989. Americans' Views on Health Care: Foolish Inconsistencies? *Health Affairs* 8: 111–12.

Hospitals. 1987. Indigent Care: Public Wants Government to Pay. 5 October, p. 152.

―――. 1989. Politics Kill Indigent Care "Sin" Tax and Lottery. 5 September, p. 70.

Intergovernmental Health Policy Project. 1988. *Major Changes in State Medicaid and Indigent Care Projects, 1988*. Washington, DC: Intergovernmental Health Policy Project, George Washington University.

Jones, Katherine R. 1989. The Florida Health Care Access Act: A Blended Regulatory/ Competitive Approach to the Indigent Care Problem. *Journal of Health Politics, Policy and Law* 14: 261–85.

Medical Benefits. 1989. Small Business Will Choose Layoffs, Shutdowns if Forced to Offer Health Benefits. 6: 4.

Monheit, Alan C., et al. 1985. The Employed Uninsured and the Role of Public Policy. *Inquiry* 22: 349.

Moyer, M. Eugene. 1989. Data Watch: A Revised Look at the Number of Uninsured Americans. *Health Affairs* 8 (Summer): 102–10.

Reinhardt, Uwe. 1984. The Problem of "Uncompensated Care," or Are Americans Really as Mean as They Look? In *Proceedings—Uncompensated Care in a Competitive Environment: Whose Problem is It?* Washington, DC: Department of Health and Human Services.

Robert Wood Johnson Foundation. 1987. *Access to Health Care in the United States: Results of a 1986 Survey*. Princeton, NJ: Robert Wood Johnson Foundation.

Short, Pamela Farley, et al. 1989. Profile of Uninsured Americans (National Medical Expenditure Survey Research Findings 1). Washington, DC: Department of Health and Human Services, DHHS Pub. No. (PHS) 89-3443.

Thorpe, Kenneth E., et al. 1989. Including the Poor: The Fiscal Impacts of Medicaid Expansion. *Journal of the American Medical Association* 261: 1003–7.

U.S. General Accounting Office. 1989. *Health Insurance: An Overview of the Working Uninsured*. Washington, DC: GAO.

The Deconstructed Center:
Of Policy Plagues on Political Houses

Lawrence D. Brown

The problems of the disadvantaged groups addressed in this special issue share several troubling features. They are serious. They have (in most cases) worsened over the 1980s. They have been met by modest governmental efforts at amelioration at best, by retrenchment at worst. They show no signs of withering away in the 1990s under the impact of market or other nonpublic cures. As we enter the 1990s, significant numbers of elderly and disabled cannot afford humane long-term-care settings and services. Morbidity and mortality among lower-income infants and children remain depressingly high by cross-national standards. Hundreds of thousands of Americans are homeless, and millions are hungry. Preventive and educational efforts against AIDS and public support for the chronic care of people who have contracted the disease remain halting. Drug addiction, apparently immune of late to a cyclical downturn in abuse that should have set in years ago, plagues the streets and crowds the courts and jails. Mental health policy presupposes community capacities for counseling and treatment that have not been adequately realized. Roughly 15 percent of the nonaged population lacks health insurance coverage.

The rational optimist in most of us believes in some reliable connection between problem stimuli and public responses. If social conditions become "sufficiently" tragic, governmental empathies and energies will somehow, eventually, get mobilized. What then accounts for the stubborn disconnections between problems and politics for more than a decade?

An explanation might lie in the realm of culture: perhaps the American value system, so severely moralistic in judging the poor and so impervious to the moral claims of the welfare state, is the source of immobilism. The importance of cultural peculiarities can never be discounted in U.S. social policy, but they can illuminate only part of the story. For one thing, the United States *has* embraced a range of welfare state programs that, though highly incomplete by European standards, are extensive and expensive nonetheless. Second, American social politics are erratic in ways that culture—presumably by definition—is not. We have our ups (the 1930s and 1960s) and our downs (the 1950s and 1980s). Something must surely be added to bedrock cultural variables to explain the lowly standing of the 1980s on the activism index. Finally, opinion polls, ambiguous and unreliable though they often are, seem to challenge the premise: respondents often assert a fairly high degree of sympathy—at least at a general level—for many of the disadvantaged, and assert that they wish to see their problems addressed.

A second explanation could be structural: the intermittent (usually chronic) deadlock and stalemate that now afflict policymaking simply amount to non-business as usual. American separation of powers, federalism, and extensive private clout are all famous for checking political action despite strong popular demands for it. Executive branch ideology notwithstanding, however, the 1980s saw considerable activism in federal health policy. Government revised Medicare payments to hospitals by enacting a prospective payment system in 1983 and then changed Medicare reimbursement for physicians by adopting resource-based relative value scales in 1989. Federal legislation also made small but significant enlargements in Medicaid, mandated continued health insurance options for laid-off workers and others, and tried (abortively) to introduce new catastrophic benefits into Medicare. By no means paralyzed in the 1980s, the federal government showed itself capable of rapid, decisive action, when it chose to exert itself—the proviso that, of course, simply restates the question with which we set out.

Perhaps the disconnection between problems and politics reflects a deeper disjunction between social ends and policy means. A society that in principle wants to respond to the needs of the disadvantaged might not agree either on just what it wants to tell government to do or that government should be encouraged to exercise in this sphere the discretion it has used on other occasions to advance other causes (notably cost containment and revenue-neutral extensions of benefits). Inferences from polls supporting initiatives for the disadvantaged (or expressing dissatisfaction with the system in general) of a mandate for governmental activism may rest on a large non sequitur, for the public may "want" change yet lack confidence that government will deliver it wisely and fairly. The first condition, uncertainty about fashioning means to ends, suggests that general sympathies may conceal an underlying ambivalence that is more analytical ("diagnostic," so to speak) than cultural—namely, uncertainty about whether the social problems at which new governmental efforts would aim are amenable to improvement by any practical set of public (or other) interventions. The second condition, unwillingness to insist that government exercise discretion and get on with the specialized tasks of policymaking in the absence of clear popular agreement on what should be done, suggests that the narrow confines of 1980s activism within legislative stratagems that either save or circumvent new federal outlays may harbor a profound failure of political trust. This essay argues that the conjunction of these two factors—the rise of "diagnostic" uncertainty about the disadvantaged and the decline of political trust in government as a problem-solving force—largely explains the disjunction between problems and policies illustrated repeatedly in this special issue.

The proximate origins of these inhibiting forces go back about 25 years to the launching of the War on Poverty in 1964-65. Between 1964 and 1968 the federal government, under the leadership of Lyndon Johnson and a Democratic Congress, enacted wide-ranging federal interventions in civil rights, health, housing, manpower training, education, law enforcement, and other arenas. Much was promised, more implied: the public was given to expect that new programs would generate better race relations, lower or more slowly growing welfare spending, better education and job skills among the poor, and lower crime—in short, a "Great Society." Within five years, results stood sharply at odds with projections: blacks were rioting in the inner cities, and racial separatism was gaining adherents; crime and drug use increased; welfare spending rose and family breakups accelerated; and the problems of the "underclass" refused to yield to the federal assault. Meanwhile, anger over the war in Vietnam further destabilized domestic politics. In 1968 Johnson declined to seek renomination in that year's presidential election, which sent Richard Nixon to the White House.

Within four years, a liberal hour had turned into what would become a conservative epoch. By 1970 conservative theorists had thrown down four challenges to liberalism that went, and remain today, largely unanswered. First, neo-conservatives, influenced by research such as the report on *Equality of Educational Opportunity* by James Coleman and his colleagues and the growing body of political science studies of implementation, took to the pages of *The Public Interest* and other journals to belabor the inability of the federal government to set realistic goals and to bewail its addiction to "throwing money at problems." Second, in 1968 Edward C. Banfield presented a powerful (albeit speculative and controversial) explanation of this alleged federal futility: government problem solving failed for largely cultural reasons. That is, it could do little to change the outlook and behavior of thousands of lower-class people imbued with a present-oriented time horizon and no capacity (or will) to respond to the new, improved "objective opportunities" government preferred. Third, in a 1970 book entitled *The Real Majority*, Richard M. Scammon and Ben J. Wattenberg postulated the social consequences of the turmoil surrounding new government programs. They discerned broad indignation over "the social issue," a sense among the real majority of average and forgotten Americans that liberal politicians, bureaucrats, and social engineers were provoking an impressionable lower class to violate basic norms of order, civility, and acceptable public deportment. Increasingly, the middle class laid at liberal doors the crime, drug abuse, and racial tension that thrived when blacks and the poor were (supposedly) encouraged to abuse the system that (supposedly) abused them. Fourth, Kevin Phillips projected the political consequences of the social issue, namely, "the emerging Republican majority" (the title of his 1969 book), exemplified by the 57 percent of voters who supported Richard Nixon or George Wallace in the 1968 presidential race. Disgusted by liberal policies, traditional Democratic voters in the South, the suburbs, and elsewhere had become available to the Republicans not as intermittent defectors (as in 1956) but as durable supporters. These four challenges embodied a thicket of analytical and political complications that policymaking for the disadvantaged would henceforth have to clear to regain legitimacy.

If one extrapolates the political scientists' famous 36-year cycle, the election of 1968 should have brought a "critical realignment," a shift of popular loyalties between the two major parties of a size, clarity, and duration sufficient to tilt the balance of governing power from the Democrats to the Republicans. For whatever reason, the returns were mixed: Nixon won, but narrowly, over Hubert Humphrey, and both houses of Congress stayed under Democratic control. But the shifts Phillips described in 1969 were unmistakable in Nixon's landslide victory over George McGovern in 1972. Watergate then intervened to scramble the signals for the rest of the decade. The three presidential races in the 1980s, however, restored and confirmed the earlier ambiguous pattern as Republicans won resounding presidential victories despite continuing Democratic predominance in Congress. Realignment or no (an issue for other audiences, occasions, and authors), the 20-year record between 1968 and 1988 shows that Republicans have held the White House for 16 of 20 years; that in five of six presidential contests voters selected the more conservative candidate; and that the dominant conservative of the 1980s (Reagan) stood markedly to the right of his 1970s counterpart (Nixon). More is at work here than such incidental Democratic misfortunes as Jimmy Carter endured with inflation, OPEC, and Iran. Republican conservatives may not have won a clear critical realignment in partisan terms, but they certainly seem to have achieved a rightward ideological realignment in the policy realm.

Part of the explanation lies in the failure of Great Society liberalism, especially its inability convincingly to rebut the major elements of the conservative critique of the late 1960s, and, indeed, its frequently lofty refusal to try to fashion a rebuttal. Yet liberals do owe a quizzical public an accounting for the rising social budgets, worsening race relations, soaring crime, and the rest, all quite the opposite of what was supposed to follow in the wake of new exertions by big government. To a public persuaded that Washington haphazardly "throws money at problems," it avails little to reply, as some liberals do, that all would have been well if only more had been spent. Moreover, Great Society liberalism remains highly vulnerable to Banfield's cultural critique because so many programs (Medicare is the main exception), influenced by sociological theory and social work practice, aimed to break into a "cycle of poverty" by educating disadvantaged children, improving job skills, promoting community empowerment, and other strategies that presupposed unproven "technologies" for changing behavior. To dismiss as "blaming the victim" skeptical queries about why federally enhanced "objective opportunities" did not produce the expected middle-classification of the lower orders is condescending and impolitic.

By the mid-1970s it was clear to anyone not entirely tone deaf to popular sentiment that the social issue had become a powerful if inchoate political force. As urban riots and campus depredations subsided, "crime in the streets" took center stage. The old dichotomy of "deserving" and "undeserving" poor was complicated by a new entrant, the "predatory" poor, who seemed far more menacing than the organized (and therefore more disciplined) mob syndicates and juvenile gangs that worried the populace in the 1950s and 1960s. Liberals often responded to fears of the predatory poor—a group of fundamental importance to the politics of policy toward the disadvantaged then and still—by insisting that law and order were "code words for racism" (directed, of course, at "victims" unjustly "blamed" for mugging and murdering others mainly of their own class and race). Battered badly by the crime issue, liberals in the 1990s cannot hope to cross the threshold of legitimacy and regain a modicum of political trust until they recognize that for many Americans the hungry, homeless, mentally ill, and addicted are viewed as prime exemplars of the predatory poor, and until they acknowledge that law and order is both the first obligation a state owes its citizens and a crucial corrective to the Hobbesian state of nature into which many Americans believe their society has degenerated.

Liberals' astounding incompetence at demonstrating that government programs are more than bottomless pits for taxpayers' money, at moving debate from the shifting sands of behavioral change to the firmer ground of income maintenance and family financial assistance, and at calming and protecting society by insisting that victims who victimize deserve both blame and punishment has contributed massively to the consolidation and extension of the emerging Republican ideological majority. Barring fortuitous windfalls from economic downturns, foreign imbroglios, domestic scandals, or other bad luck on the Republican watch, the Democrats are unlikely to find a broader constituency until they develop a newly responsive social philosophy that salves public sensibilities that liberal slights have helped to rub raw. And without such a social philosophy supported by a broader liberal Democratic constituency, there is little hope for new policy departures for the disadvantaged.

Two decades of conservative "progress" are not, however, explained by liberal failings alone. Conservatives themselves, especially since 1980, deserve a large share of the "credit" for astutely and aggressively exploiting liberal weaknesses. The decline of political trust was not lost on the Nixonites, who knew well whereof Phillips spoke, and the sour rhetorical forays of Spiro

Agnew (whom Eugene McCarthy dubbed "Nixon's Nixon") tried to speed the Republican emergence by inflaming the social issue. But although Nixon surely included "the Establishment" among his myriad visceral dislikes, he was far too much the respectable Establishment figure to pull out all stops in discrediting the government in which he had long served and which he now headed in tumultuous times. Remarkably responsible (especially when contrasted with coming attractions), the Nixon team set out, under the guidance of Daniel P. Moynihan, Richard Nathan, and others, to distinguish analytically the proper respective roles of the private sector, the states, and the federal government. Nor did they refuse to follow arguments that prescribed new federal duties, such as the Family Assistance Plan, proposed and nearly won in the early 1970s, and federal leadership in promoting health maintenance organizations.

In retrospect, the Nixon years appear to have been less a safety valve that allowed steam to escape from the social issue than an inconclusive intermission in which that issue continued to build explosive pressure released in part in the 1980s but far from spent today. With the Reagan years there arrived an end to responsible conservatism and a new demogogic indulgence in the scarcely constrained exploitation of social suspicion and political distrust. Reagan unabashedly portrayed the federal government as the root of most evils and the purveyor of misconceived programs that only served to spoil individual character and depress capital accumulation; depleted the federal revenue base by insisting that the tax dollars liberals would throw at problems rest undisturbed in the wallet of the taxpayer; recklessly embraced huge budget deficits as a brake on policy activism; and promoted a mindless market worship as the one true policy faith. Perceiving how generalized social resentments might, with more than a little simplistic rhetorical encouragement, congeal into a focused attack on government and taxes themselves, the Reaganites proceeded to invoke the ensuing budget shortfalls as the instant all-purpose rebuttal to the claims of the disadvantaged.

Accepting realities they could not change, liberals adroitly improvised activist stratagems in the 1980s, notably the creative resort to revenue-neutral expansions (new options in Medicaid, for example, were offset against savings projected from cost containment schemes), mandates that imposed the costs of public decisions on private actors (the requirement that employers offer continued health insurance coverage to laid-off workers and others at group rates but at individual expense, and new civil rights protections for the disabled), and self-financing for new benefits (the addition of catastrophic coverage to Medicare in 1988). Given the relative paucity of savings offsets, the first strategy can be incremental and marginal at best, while the second is increasingly stymied by private sector resistance to the growth of costly government mandates, and, as vividly illustrated by the unceremonious repeal of the catastrophic benefits in 1989, the third has less promise than initially assumed. The limits of the improvisations of the 1980s serve to leave on every pair of honest lips in 1990 the possibility that new taxes may be needed to meet the needs of the disadvantaged. The conventional wisdom, however, powerfully reinforced by the fate of candid candidate Walter Mondale in 1984, is that such honesty is the best policy for political suicide.

Ronald Reagan's two terms and the succession of his heir George Bush have decisively sundered the ever-tenuous American links between political success and policy substance. A responsible conservatism would take a hard line on crime—and cash in some of the legitimacy and trust thus acquired on new benefits for the disadvantaged. It would delude neither itself nor the public about the "magic" of a marketplace that does not raise all ships and can, if blindly indulged, drown the poorest of the poor. It would maintain a pragmatic if skeptical attitude toward government and would continue, not abandon, the Nixonian quest for defensible distinctions among the roles of sectors of society and levels of government.

Above all, a responsible conservatism would join a newly responsive liberalism (responsive, that is, to the concerns of "middle America") in distinguishing among the several worlds of the disadvantaged and in drawing out the highly diverse policy implications of their topographies. Some of the poor can indeed be effectively assisted by economic growth (or tax cuts that allow them to keep more of their low incomes). For them, Reaganomics may be a sound prescription. But some poor need to have money "thrown" at their problems—the lower-income elderly or people with AIDS who cannot afford decent chronic care, mothers and children facing financial obstacles to preventive and primary care, those who endure hunger because their pay (or food stamps) will not stretch to cover decent meals each day, those who haunt the streets because they cannot raise the rent, addicts seeking treatment and cure, lower-income workers who need help to buy health insurance. These are the saddest casualties of the 1980s, for they are in a very direct causal sense victims of misguided policy, of missed opportunities and undiscerning cutbacks.

Some poor are culturally "disturbed" but not incorrigible. These—some drug abusers, homeless, mentally ill, and others—require the fabled integrated networks of social and medical services—outreach, counseling, treatment, monitoring, and more—that are not only costly and labor-intensive but are also beyond the bureaucratic capacities of most local governments. For this group, subsidies and entitlements often must be supplemented by excursions into the poorly charted waters of behavioral change. Finally, some disadvantaged unhappily do fall into the ranks of the culturally incorrigible. These are individuals so unbalanced or amoral as to lie beyond the reach of general economic progress, targeted programs of financial or in-kind assistance, or intensive local social services. For the pacific members of this group, there is little good that policy can do. For the malignant—career criminals and predators, a subgroup of unknown but far from negligible size—society's proper response is law enforcement: deterrence, detection, detention. The multiple worlds of the disadvantaged and their heterogeneous policy correlates demand new synthetic blends of principle and pragmatism that today's irresponsible conservatives and unresponsive liberals seem unable to fathom, let alone fashion.

Legend has long held that the United States is the classic home of the pragmatic political center—in Hartz's terms, the cultural "fragment" that left true Left and true Right behind in Europe and nourished instead an unchallenged bourgeois Lockean liberalism, massively stable albeit mightily stifling. While European nations battled within and among themselves over various polar "isms," America held effortlessly and contentedly to the center. Whatever its past merits, this comparative image is a doubtful guide to the realities of today's partisan politics. And party competition aside, the image fails badly as an account of the contemporary politics of policy.

Over the last 25 years, which have so unsettled the U.S. policy debate, Western European—and, it now appears, Eastern European—nations have worked to reconcile capitalist economic structures with broad social welfare programs. Most have found some form of *soziale Marktwirtschaft* (German for the "social market state") appealing and workable. Virtually all recognize—as Reaganite conservatives never have—that in a capitalist society the scope of the state should vary directly, not inversely, with the scope of the market: the wider the sphere of market activities, the bigger the government needed to contain and constrain various messes that do not self-correct in a laissez-faire regime and that, left unattended, threaten to dissolve capitalist legitimacy in ceaseless waves of boom and bust. This creative, constructive centrism has largely eluded the United States, which gyrates between a liberalism unattuned to powerful public sensibilities and a conservatism ensconced in a fantasyland of privatistic "solutions."

The American policy center has ceased to hold, has largely faded from view. Its reconstruction awaits the invention of a new Burkean liberalism, committed to social justice and reform, but mindful and respectful of expectations and norms honored by the legions of real, average, and forgotten middle Americans. It equally awaits a new Benthamite conservatism, devoted to preserving private rights and liberties against encroaching government but courageous and honest in facing facts squarely, in refusing to trivialize the tragedy of policy paralysis for the disadvantaged with incantations to the myths and magic of the marketplace.

Epilogue: Tales of Trouble

James A. Morone

Taken together, the preceding chapters are a gloomy read. Across the jumble of topics—organized by disease, deprivation, and age group—we get a consistent message: These Americans are doing badly, and, for most, things are getting worse. But what do the tales of trouble add up to? Consider four different stories that this volume tells.

First, here are snapshots of disadvantage that reflect poorly on the Reagan domestic policies—what might be called tales of churlishness. Thus, Lipsky and Thibodeau note the "churning" of food stamp recipients: reducing expenditures by arbitrarily denying claims (and waiting for the recipients to appeal) or fiddling with the bureaucratic forms (and waiting till they figure them out). Vladeck pictures a cowardly response to homelessness. And disabled Americans, to recall an instance not discussed above, were forced to sue for benefits, one at a time, even after their district courts had ruled other plaintiffs in the same circumstances eligible. (The restrictive policy framed by the Department of Health and Human Services was known as "non-acquiescence.")

This mean season opened with a systematic theory. As Charles Murray (1984) articulated it, government programs harmed the poor. His view has no allies here. Interestingly, there is not even much urge to take the argument on. These articles do not debate the Reagan policies; they simply chart the deleterious consequences. Moreover, they largely share the view that we are grappling with the problem of political stalemate rather than with puzzles which are intrinsically difficult to resolve. While AIDS or drug abuse may trouble policymakers across the industrialized world, no other nation faces, say, gaps in health insurance coverage anything like ours. The problem does not require deep thinking, suggests Larry Brown, until one ponders how to weld a political coalition which might address it (at which point, he implies, deep thinking evaporates into despair). Similarly, homelessness, hunger, and childhood poverty await political coalitions more than policy conceptions. The problem has been reversed: from the public sector's imperialism, which Murray lambasted, to its impasse, which we now lament.

This story puts us on reassuringly familiar political ground. After all, the tension between active and passive government, between "the house of Have and the house of Want," has defined the difference between liberals and conservatives for over a century (Schlesinger 1945). Liberals find the long view reassuring, for they often detect alternating cycles of liberal and conservative ascendancy (Schlesinger 1986; Burnham 1970). The activism of the Progressives, the New Dealers, and the Great Society alternated with the relative quiescence of the late 1910s and 1920s, the late 1940s and 1950s, the 1970s and 1980s. Such broad generalizations may be perilous (each of the "conservative" eras saw ostensibly "liberal" innovations), but that has not checked speculation about a new leftward swing. (See the essays in *The American Prospect* [1990] for a striking illustration.) Does this volume offer any intimations of an emerging political realignment? Indeed, what would that evidence look like? The questions introduce a second, more subtle story running through the preceding chapters.

The essays testify that pluralism is alive and well in policy analysis. Future changes are generally predicted (and past changes often explained) by the motion of groups as they enter and exit coalitions. Child policy features the odd alliance of liberals and right-to-lifers. AIDS politics turns on the troubled relations between gay, Latino, and African-American communities. Health insurance politics features the elaborate posturing of business coalitions (with their deliciously ironic call for government action now that compulsory employer action looms as an alternative); however, business leaders are not likely to agree with one another, much less with potentially sympathetic providers or politicians. Therefore, we are advised to expect no action. Perhaps coalitions figure so prominently because, as Larry Brown suggests, Americans do not have reliable political alternatives—responsible political parties, respected civil servants—that are likely to foster social reform.

Implicit in the pluralistic flux lies an important account of the American welfare system: redistributive programs flourish when poor beneficiaries find respectably bourgeois champions. Food stamps evolved from an agricultural surplus program and remained lodged in the Department of Agriculture. Hospitals, nursing homes, and medical societies are often Medicaid's most effective local champions. Housing for the poor operated through real estate entrepreneurs who took advantage of subsidies and tax incentives. As a mind-stretching contrast, note that after almost a decade of privatization policy, over one in five British domiciles still belong to the government.

Producer groups mobilize more easily. They evoke the constituency servicing for which both ends of Pennsylvania Avenue have grown justly famous. However, respectable clienteles offer more than powerful alliances in the scramble of American politics; policy programs that involve them project a very different—and far more politically popular—image than programs geared to the poor. It is more politic to support farmers than "welfare queens," easier to legislate tax expenditures (which operate through the hard-working entrepreneur) than to direct subsidies to poor people. The trouble, of course, is that such welfare coalitions evolve gradually, quietly, inadvertently. When they come unstuck, they are very difficult to put together again.

The job of reorganizing a social welfare coalition falls, willy-nilly, to the Democratic party. Here is the story of juggling coalitions writ large. There is a barely submerged theme running through the volume, finally brought to the surface by Larry Brown's commentary, which might be called "Waiting for the Democrats." In our mixed political era, Republicans dominate the presidency and, perhaps consequently, the national agenda; Democrats hang on in Congress, warily, defensively, without clear plan or message. Liberals seem entirely frustrated by the challenge to articulate a message that they can sustain on the hustings. Their problem, in my view, lies not merely in the content of the message but in the coalition it must mobilize. The party, as it is presently constituted, straddles the great divide of American politics: race. This is the issue on which liberal coalitions—from the Democratic party on down— come unraveled.

Race is the hidden story in this volume. In every chapter, the data create the same portrait: there is deprivation in many quarters, but "minorities" suffer a disproportionate share. Here is a potent American dilemma which is often obscured (as it is here) by the functional categories of our policy discourse. Whether the topic is poverty among the aged, the risk of homelessness among children, the incidence of drug abuse, or the raw statistical probability of ending up in jail (now approaching 3 percent for males), the portrait of black America that leaks out of collections such as this is extraordinarily grim.

Moreover, American racial problems are enormously intricate, a long-standing mix of every issue discussed above. It is difficult to find plausible solutions or potential coalitions. When social scientists debate the cycles of American history, their arguments are about class politics—movements for and against the poor and working classes. There is no comforting analogue in American race relations. On the contrary, the last Democratic ascendancy almost passed black Americans by, for it was anchored by Southern Democrats. (Thomas Dewey failed to win a single former Confederate state in 1948; Richard Nixon won only two in 1960.) The policy consequence was a long-standing reluctance to engage in racial reforms. Franklin Roosevelt would not endorse federal curbs on lynching, Harry Truman could not get his domestic agenda past the Southern Democrats, and John Kennedy sacrificed civil rights to maintain his fragile congressional majority till after the Birmingham demonstrations of 1963. When Lyndon Johnson followed Kennedy's conversion and actually won voting rights in 1964, he was presiding over the end of the old Democratic coalition. The party, which has won the White House only once since, is still looking for the way to forge a new alignment. Quadrennial Democratic squirming over the "Jesse Jackson factor" vividly demonstrates the obstinate schism that the party must overcome.

The issue lurks in every chapter of this volume. The dilemmas of the underprivileged, the dynamics of American welfare politics, and the decline of the Democrats are all powerfully tied to the American racial perplexity.

Finally, this volume speaks about America as a community. It reports on the present state of an ancient tension—that between individual and collective values, between self-interest and shared interests. Judith Feder takes up the matter directly when she speculates about the move to make the aged responsible for financing new Medicare benefits; this, she argues, will eviscerate reform in long-term care, for, as a group, the aged cannot afford it. The financing strategy is emblematic of the contemporary insurance regime, rating risk groups ever more precisely in what amounts to a broad social motion away from cross-subsidization. Those who enjoy the correlates of good health (the young, the wealthy, the educated, people who hold desirable jobs, and those who have not been seriously ill) might save themselves (and their employers) cash if they can separate themselves from their fellow citizens. In the process, the concept of shared risk—indeed, of social insurance—begins to unravel. The refusal to share resources jeopardizes our ability to address social problems.

The scramble away from shared risk is, of course, not peculiar to the 1980s. It draws on vague but potent American traditions celebrating individualism, promoting market competition, and bashing governments. In the 1980s conservative think tanks and authors molded these amorphous instincts into policy-analytic respectability; President Reagan sent them out over the airwaves with extraordinary political effect.

Perhaps free-market fancies were relevant to an earlier social order marked, as Benjamin Barber (1986: 54) put it, by "open spaces, empty jobs and unmade fortunes." However, as these papers all testify, there are heavy social consequences to pursuing the individualist idyll in a complex, interconnected, late industrial society. Still, where are the other possibilities? What other ideological traditions might Americans draw from?

Not long ago, I heard a young French Canadian unwittingly suggest an alternative: "In the American health care system," he asked a panel of health care specialists, "who worries about the people's health?" There are few hints of such a notion anywhere in this volume. Indeed, it is a conception strikingly absent from popular American discourse. What is missing is a communitarian counter to the images of individualism. Shared values, civic responsibility, and common interest have a long American heritage, too (Morone 1990). Perhaps nothing about America moved Alexis de Tocqueville (1969: 189–90) to hyperbole so much as the "improvised assembly of neighbors" that sprang to one another's assistance in times of trouble. These communities, he wrote, seemed to flow "directly from the hand of God." The comparatively quiet, often overlooked American tradition of community offers a broad philosophical alternative to the excesses of the past decade.

Over time, Americans have managed a tenuous balance between celebration of the individual and responsibility for the community, between market striving and civic sharing, between the private sphere and the public good. Individualistic values always threaten to overwhelm communitarian ones. The essays in this volume show what happens when they do.

References

American Prospect. 1990. 1 (1).

Barber, Benjamin. 1986. The Compromised Republic: Public Purposelessness in America. In *The Moral Foundations of the American Republic*, ed. Robert Horwitz. Charlottesville: University Press of Virginia.

Burnham, Walter Dean. 1970. *Critical Elections and the Mainsprings of American Politics*. New York: W. W. Norton.

Morone, James A. 1990. *The Democratic Wish: Popular Participation and the Limits of American Government*. New York: Basic Books.

Murray, Charles. 1984. *Losing Ground: American Social Policy, 1950–1980*. New York: Basic Books.

Schlesinger, Arthur M., Jr. 1945. *The Age of Jackson*. Boston: Little, Brown.

———. 1986. *The Cycles of American History*. Boston: Houghton Mifflin.

Tocqueville, Alexis de. 1969. *Democracy in America*, trans. George Lawrence, ed. J. P. Mayer. Garden City, NY: Doubleday Anchor.

Index

Contributors

Deborah A. Stone holds the David R. Pokross chair in law and social policy at the Heller School, Brandeis University. Her research blends historical, comparative, legal, and political science approaches to diverse topics in health and welfare policy. During 1985–1986, she held a Guggenheim fellowship and was a fellow in law and political science at Harvard Law School. During 1990, she was the Lester Crown Visiting Professor of Public Management in the School of Organization and Management, Yale University. In addition to numerous articles, she has written *The Limits of Professional Power: The National Health System of West Germany* (University of Chicago Press, 1980), *The Disabled State* (Temple University Press, 1984), and *Policy Paradox and Political Reason* (Scott, Foresman/Little, Brown, 1988). Her current work focuses on legal rights, new medical technologies, and health insurance. She is the senior editor of *The American Prospect* and the book review editor of *JHPPL*.

Theodore R. Marmor received his A.B. and Ph.D. degrees from Harvard University and taught at the universities of Wisconsin, Minnesota, and Chicago before coming to Yale in 1979 as chairman of the Center for Health Studies. He is currently professor of public management and political science in the Yale School of Organization and Management and Yale College. He was editor of the *Journal of Health Politics, Policy and Law* from 1980 to 1984 and is the author of *The Politics of Medicare* (Aldine, 1973) and *Political Analysis and American Medical Care* (Cambridge University Press, 1983). He writes and lectures frequently about the politics of the welfare state. Most recently he coedited (with Jerry Mashaw) and contributed to *Social Security: Beyond the Rhetoric of Crisis*, published by Princeton University Press in 1988, and, with Mashaw and Philip Harvey, has just completed *America's Misunderstood Welfare State* (Basic Books, 1990). Dr. Marmor served as special assistant to HEW's Commission on Income Maintenance Programs from 1968 to 1970 and on the Presidential Commission on a National Agenda for the 1980s. In 1987–1988 he was a fellow of the Russell Sage Foundation, and in 1987 he was named the first American fellow of the Canadian Institute for Advanced Research.

Judith Feder, Ph.D., co-director of the Center for Health Policy Studies, Georgetown University, was staff director of the Pepper Commission (U.S. Bipartisan Commission on Comprehensive Health Care). She is a political scientist who has written extensively on a broad range of health and long-term-care policy issues: the implementation of Medicare, the adequacy of public and private health insurance for the elderly, financing of long-term care, alternative designs for national health insurance, provider payment strategies, and hospitals' delivery of care to the poor. Dr. Feder received her M.A. and Ph.D. in political science from Harvard University and her B.A. from Brandeis University. Prior to taking up her position at Georgetown University, she served as a senior research associate at the Urban Institute for seven years.

Alice Sardell is an associate professor in the Department of Urban Studies at Queens College of the City University of New York. She received a Ph.D. in politics from New York University, where she was a DHEW fellow in political science and health policy. Her broad research interests are in the politics of social policy. She has published articles on the welfare rights movement, the politics of primary health care, and health policy in New York state. She is a coeditor of *Critical Issues in Health Policy* (Lexington Books, 1981) and the author of *The U.S. Experiment in Social Medicine: The Community Health Center Program, 1965–1986* (University of Pittsburgh Press, 1988), which discusses the political history of the federally supported community health center program during two decades, within the context of an analysis of primary health care policy in the U.S. She is currently examining managed care as a strategy for providing primary health care services to low-income residents of New York state.

Bruce C. Vladeck has been president of the United Hospital Fund of New York since 1983. He also serves on the Prospective Payment ,ssessment Commission and on numerous other boards and commissions at the national, state, and local level. Prior to joining the United Hospital Fund, Dr. Vladeck served as assistant vice-president of the Robert Wood Johnson Foundation and as assistant commissioner for health planning and resources development of the New Jersey State Department of Health. Previously, he taught at Columbia University. Dr. Vladeck has lectured and written extensively on issues of health care policy, health care financing, and long-term care. He is the author of *Unloving Care: The Nursing Home Tragedy* and of numerous articles and book chapters. He received his B.A. from Harvard and his M.A. and Ph.D. in political science from the University of Michigan.

Michael Lipsky is professor of political science at the Massachusetts Institute of Technology. His research has focused on political strategies of relatively powerless groups, on police, schools, welfare offices, and other public-service bureaucracies, on the politics of nonprofit organization, and on hunger and homelessness in the United States. Books he has written include *Protest on City Politics, Commission Politics: The Processing of Racial Crisis in America*, and *Street-Level Bureaucracy*.

Marc A. Thibodeau received his J.D. from Boston College Law School and an S.M. from the Massachusetts Institute of Technology, where he studied international and domestic agriculture and nutrition policy. He currently works for the legal division of the Massachusetts Department of Public Welfare, where he represents the commonwealth in administrative and judicial proceedings against the Food and Nutrition Service of the U.S. Department of Agriculture and the U.S. Department of Health and Human Services. With Michael Lipsky, he has coauthored "Feeding the Hungry with Surplus Commodities" (*American Political Science Quarterly*, Summer 1988), "Delivery of Federal Food Assistance: Twenty Years' Experience" (prepared for the National Neighborhood Coalition conference, November 1985), "Food in the Warehouses, Hunger in the Streets: A Report of the Temporary Emergency Food Assistance Program" (MIT, July 1985), and "Dilemmas of Utilizing Voluntary Organizations for Public Purposes" (prepared for the annual meeting of the American Political Science Association, 1984).

Daniel M. Fox, Ph.D., is president of the Milbank Memorial Fund. Until 1989 he was professor of humanities in medicine and director of the Center for Assessing Health Services at the State University of New York at Stony Brook. He holds A.B., A.M., and Ph.D. degrees in history from Harvard University, where he taught before coming to Stony Brook in 1971. He has also served in Massachusetts state government and on the staff of several federal agencies. He has written numerous articles on public policy, the history of medicine, health affairs, and photography. His books include the prize-winning *The Discovery of Abundance* (1967), *Economists and Health Care* (1979), *Health Politics, Health Policies: The Experience of Britain and America, 1911 – 1965* (1986), and (with Christopher Lawrence) *Photographing Medicine: Images and Power in Britain and America since 1840* (1988). He coedited and contributed to *AIDS The Burdens of History* (1988) and *Financing Health Care for Persons with AIDS: The First Studies, 1985 – 88.*

William E. McAuliffe is an associate professor in the Department of Psychiatry, Harvard Medical School at Cambridge Hospital, and a lecturer in the Department of Behavioral Sciences at the Harvard School of Public Health. He received his doctorate in sociology from the Johns Hopkins University. His research has focused on drug abuse and general health policy, planning, and regulation, especially with regard to methodological issues. He has recently completed a drug abuse treatment plan for Rhode Island. He and his staff have developed a program for treating cocaine addiction, Recovery Training and Self Help. He is currently the principal investigator of a randomized trial testing the efficacy of this program. He is also principal investigator of a study of the effectiveness of street outreach and recovery programs for preventing the spread of AIDS among intravenous drug users.

Kathleen Ackerman is an assistant to William McAuliffe, an associate professor in the Department of Psychiatry, Harvard Medical School at Cambridge Hospital. She is currently helping Dr. McAuliffe prepare and edit a revised edition of a manual for the aftercare of recovering drug addicts. She received her bachelor of arts degree in government from Wesleyan University. She will enter New York University Law School in 1991 to study and eventually teach American legal history.

M. Gregg Bloche is associate professor of law at the Georgetown University Law Center and co-director of the Georgetown—Johns Hopkins joint degree program in law and public health. He received his J.D. and M.D. from Yale University and recently completed a residency in psychiatry at the Columbia-Presbyterian Medical Center. While a resident, he was also a lecturer in law at Columbia. His current research interests are medical cost containment, mental health policy, and international human rights.

Francine Cournos is associate clinical professor of psychiatry at Columbia University's College of Physicians and Surgeons, director of Columbia's Washington Heights Community Service, and consultant to the New York State Office of Mental Health on public policy issues. She has written, lectured, and consulted on clinical and policy issues in community psychiatry.

Lawrence D. Brown is professor and head of the Division of Health Policy and Management in the School of Public Health at Columbia University. He has served on the faculty of the University of Michigan and the staff of the Brookings Institution. Brown writes on the competitive and regulatory issues in health policy and on the politics of health care policy-making more generally. He is currently (with Catherine McLaughlin) evaluating the Robert Wood Johnson Foundation's community programs for affordable health care and its program for the medically uninsured.

James A. Morone is associate professor of political science at Brown University and a visiting professor of politics at the Yale School of Organization and Management. He has written extensively on the politics of health care, focusing on such issues as planning, regulation, state-level innovation, DRGs, bureaucracy, and the nature of the policy process. Professor Morone is the current editor of *JHPPL*. His recent book, *The Democratic Wish*, which appeared in the fall of 1990 (Basic Books), examines citizen participation movements and their effects throughout American history.